Laughter:
The Drug of Choice

Other books by author:

The First Humorously Medical Dictionary
(A Comical Compendium of Therapeutics)

Jest Desserts
(Of Cincinnati's 50 Plus)

Laughter:
The Drug of Choice

Definitive Doses of the Best Medicine

FOURTH EDITION

Written, Compiled and Edited by
Nicholas Hoesl, R.Ph.

LaughterDoc Publications
5745 Glow Court
Cincinnati, Ohio 45238

Laughter: The Drug of Choice
Definitive Doses of the Best Medicine

Copyright © 2013 by Nicholas Hoesl
Fourth Edition

Printed in the United States of America by
United Graphics, Inc. • Mattoon, IL
www.unitedgraphicsinc.com

ISBN: 978-0-615-76731-4

Foreword
(But not too forward)

Let's get serious…for a moment.

"Laughter — along with faith, hope, love, creativity and the will-to-live — can be regarded as an important resource in any strategy of health recovery, or, indeed, in prompting good health." This is Norman Cousins powerful prescription as author of *Anatomy of an Illness*. Because laughter is the best medicine, I want to be a part of this joy ride.

Humor and laughter reduces the level of stress hormones, perks up the immune system, relaxes muscles, clears the respiratory tract, increases circulation and eases perceived pain. If you have doubts about these claims, I encourage you to consult the latest findings in research journals. Scientists are discovering more and more conclusive evidence that our bodies hurt only when we don't laugh.

In my first book *The First Humorously Medical Dictionary* I stated that "our five senses are incomplete without the sixth, a sense of humor." Many of those early gems can be found here. Since then I have earned an M.D. (Mirth Dispenser), Pill of the Year Award and I have also become a Certified Laughter Leader, blessed with the best of therapy.

You'll find this book full of wordplay and humorous high-jinks. As a pharmacist I poke fun at my own kind as well as other health professionals. If I missed anyone, let me know.

Just as one man's mold is another man's medicine, I've kept the fun in dysfunctional. Synonyms may appear throughout to perpetuate the element of surprise. If you prefer to gather all material from same definition, refer to the contents section. Some of the text is silly, because even the poet Sophocles enjoyed a silly story with his philosophy.

Definitions and comments by yours truly are followed by an abbreviated (N.H.). Other works whose authorship is known are acknowledged.

About the use of the so-called Addendumbs. This is my smart-alecky way of adding my two cents worth, and also of speaking through the ages with the sages.

By reading this you have given me a brief control of your mind, but what I'm really after is your laughter.

N.H.

WARNING

(To be forewarned is to be for armed.)

Be aware that the new drugs found in this book, including laughter, have not been reviewed by the FDA as safe and effective.

Laughter: The Drug of Choice
Definitive Doses of the Best Medicine

FOURTH EDITION

Written, Compiled and Edited by
Nicholas Hoesl, R.Ph.

To Ginny. Keith and Linda,
who have also taught me how to be serious.

Contents
(not contentious)

AAAAA 1
AAADD 1
ABDOMINAL
  (also Indigestion) 1
ACNE VULGARIS 1
ACUPUNCTURE 2
ADDICT
  (also Drug Abuse) 2
ADVERTISING 2
AEROSOLS 3
AGING
  (also Geriatrics, Old) 3
AIDS 4
ALCOHOLIC
  (also Drunk) 4
ALCOHOLICS ANON 4
ALLERGY (also Pollen) 5
ALZHEIMER'S
  (also Senility) 5
AMNESIA 6
ANATOMY 6
ANESTHESIA 7
ANGER 7
ANOREXIA 8
ANTABUSE 8
ANTIBIOTICS
  (also Penicillin) 8
APATHY 8
APHRODISIAC 9
APOTHECARY
  (also Drugstore) 9
APPENDIX 9
ARTERY (Art) 9
ARTHRITIS 10
ATONIC
  (also Drink, Prosit) 10
AUTOINTOXICATION 11
AUTOPSY 11
BACTERIA 11
BALDNESS
  (also Hair, Toupee) 12
BANDAGE 12

BEAUTY
  (also Cosmetics) 13
BEER BELLY 14
BEDPAN 14
BELLADONNA 14
BERIBERI 15
BIRTH CONTROL (also Pill) 15
BISEXUAL 15
BLIND 16
BLOOD PRESSURE
  (also Circulation) 16
BODY DONATION 16
BODY PIERCING 17
BOTOX
  (also Wrinkles) 17
BRAIN 17
BREAST IMPLANTS
  (also Silicones) 18
BRONCHOCILATOR
  (Horsing Around) 18
BUCCAL 18
BULLDOZER
  (also Vet) 19
CANCER 19
CARDIAC ARREST
  (Gambling) 19
CATASTROPHE
  (also Pets) 20
CELEBRITY WORSHIP 20
CHIGGER 21
CHIROPRACTOR 21
CHOLESTEROL 21
CIRCULATION
  (also Blood Pressure) 21
CLAUSTROPHOBIA
  (Christmas) 22
CLOWN
  (also Comedic) 22
COCAINE 23
COCKTAIL PARTY 24
COFFEE 24
COLD 24

COLD REMEDY 25
COLON
(also Proctologist) 25
COLOSSAL.................................... 26
COMEDIC
(also Clown) 26
COMMUNICATION.................... 27
COMPUTER FATIGUE................ 27
COMPUTER VIRUS..................... 27
COMPUTER DEAF 28
CONDOM..................................... 28
CONSTIPATION
(also Laxity, Stool) 28
COSMETICS
(also Beauty)................................ 29
COUGH 29
COUNTER IRRITANT 30
CRABS 30
CRIME... 30
CRYOTHERAPY 31
DANCE THERAPY
(also Podiatry) 31
DATING
(also Dope, Liquidate) 32
DEATH
(also Dying, Epitaph) 33
DENTIST
(also Sorghum) 33
DEPRESSION 34
DERMATOLOGIST
(also Skin).................................... 34
DIABETES..................................... 35
DIAGNOSE
(also Nostalgia) 35
DIAGNOSIS.................................. 35
DIAGNOSTIC............................... 36
DIARRHEA 36
DIET 36
DIETER 37
DIGITALIS 37
DISEASE.. 37
DISEASES...................................... 38
DIURETICS
(also Kidney, Urology) 39
DOCTOR....................................... 39
DOCTOR'S LIFE 40
DOCTOR'S ORDERS.................... 40
DOCTOR TYPES 41

DOPAMINE
(also Dating)................................. 41
DRINKING
(also Atonic, Prosit) 41
DRUNKARDS
(also Alcoholics, Indulge).............. 42
DRUG ABUSE............................... 43
DRUG BUST 43
DRUG COMBINATIONS 43
DRUG NAMES 43
DRUG NAMES RENEW 44
DRUG SALES REP......................... 44
DRUGSTORE
(also Apothecary).......................... 45
DRUG TESTING 45
DYING
(also Death, Epitaph).................... 46
EGOTIST....................................... 46
ELECTROCARDIOGRAM 47
EMOTION 47
ENEMA
(also Laxity) 47
ENVIRONMENT.......................... 48
EPILEPSY....................................... 48
EPITAPH
(also Death, Dying) 48
ERECTION 49
ERECT DYSFUNCTION 49
ETHNOBOTONY 49
EXERCISE 49
EYESIGHT 50
FAMILIARITY 51
FASHION 52
FATIGUE....................................... 52
FEVER 53
FIRST AID..................................... 53
FLABBERGASTED 54
FLATULENCE
(also Gastric) 54
FLEAS 55
FLU 55
FOOD
(also Nutrition)............................. 55
FOOL... 56
FOOT & MOUTH........................ 57
FOREPLAY
(also Golf) 57
FORGETFULNESS 58

FREUD 59
FRIEND 59
FRUSTRATION 60
FUN 60
FUNERAL 61
FUNERAL DIRECTOR 61
FUNGAL 62
GASTRIC
  (also Flatulence) 62
GENES 62
GERIATRICS
  (also Aging, Old) 62
GERMS 63
GINGIVITIS 63
G I SERIES (Army) 64
GLUTEUS MAXIMUS 64
GLUTTON 64
GOLD THERAPY 65
GOSSIP 65
GRAN MAL SEIZURE 65
GYNECOLOGIST 66
HAIR
  (also Baldness) 66
HALITOSIS 66
HAPPINESS 67
HEALTH 67
HEALTH ADVICE 68
HEALTH FOOD 68
HEALTH PREVENTION 68
HEART 69
HEMORRHOIDS 69
HISTORY 70
HMO 70
HOMEOPATHY 71
HOMO SAPIENS 71
HOSPITAL 72
HOSPITAL CHARTS 72
HOSPITAL GOWN 72
HOSPITALIZATION PREP 73
HUG 73
HUMOR
  (also Laughter) 73
HYPOCHONDRIAC 74
INCOMPATIBILITY 75
INDIGESTION
  (also Abdominal) 76
INDULGENT
  (also Alcoholic, Drunk) 76

INFATUATE
  (also Obesity) 76
INNUENDO 77
INSANITY 77
INSOMNIA (also Sleep) 77
INTERCOURSE 78
INTERNS 78
JOCULAR (Sports) 78
JOCK STRAP 79
KIDNEY
  (also Diuretics, Urology) 79
KIDS 80
KISS 80
LANGUAGE 81
LAUGHTER
  (also Humor) 82
LAUGHING STOCK
  (also Bulldozer, Vet.) 83
LAXITY
  (also Constipation, Stool) 83
LAZINESS 84
LIFE 85
LIFESTYLE 86
LIQUIDATE
  (also Dating, Dope) 86
LIVER 86
LOBOTOMY (also Drinking) 87
LONGEVITY
  (also Aging, Old) 87
LOVE 87
MAGIC BULLET 89
MA HUANG 89
MAMMOGRAM 89
MARIJUANA
  (also Pharmacognocist) 89
MARRIAGE 90
MASSAGE 91
MASTURBATION 91
MEDICAL BOOKS 91
MEDICAL ECONOMICS 92
MEDICAL GRAFFITI 92
MEDICAL HISTORY 92
MEDICAL RESEARCH 93
MEDICAL SPECIALIST
  (also Specialist) 93
MEDICINE CHEST 94
MEDITATION 94
MEN 95

MENTAL IMBALANCE 95
MICROBES 96
MIDDLE AGE 96
MONEY 97
MUSICAL THERAPY................... 97
NAUSEATE.................................. 99
NEUROTIC
(also Depression) 99
NEUROPHARMACOL............... 100
NICOTINES
(also Smoking, Tobacco) 100
NITROUS OXIDE 100
NOISE
(also Tinnitus) 100
NONSENSE 101
NOSTALGIA
(also Diagnose) 101
NOVELTY
(also Writing)............................. 102
NUDISTS 102
NURSE....................................... 103
NURSING 104
NUTRITION
(also Food, Psychedeli)................ 104
OBESITY
(also Infatuate)........................... 104
OBSTETRICS
(also Ovation, Pregnancy)........... 105
OLD
(also Aging, Geriatrics) 105
OPTIMIST.................................. 106
OPTOMETRISTS 107
ORGAN DONATION 107
ORTHODONTIST...................... 107
OTOLARYNGOLOGIST............ 108
OVATION
(also Obstetrics, Pregnant) 108
PACHYDERMATOLOGIST 108
PAIN.. 109
PANACEA................................... 110
PARANOIA
(also Psychiatrist) 110
PATHOLOGY............................. 110
PATIENT 111
PEDICURE................................. 112
PENICILLIN.............................. 112
PERFUME 112
PESSIMIST 112

PETS
(also Polyestrous, Vet) 113
PHARMACIST 114
PHARMACOGNOCIST
(also Marijuana)......................... 114
PHILOSOPHY............................ 114
PHLEGM 115
PHYSICAL THERAPIST............. 115
THE PILL
(also Oral Contraceptive)............ 115
PILLAGE.................................... 116
PILL DRILL 116
PLACEBO................................... 117
PLASTIC SURGERY 117
PMS... 118
PODIATRY 118
POLLEN
(also Allergy).............................. 119
POLYESTROUS
(also Pets, Veterinarian).............. 119
POTIONS 119
PRAYER
(also Religion) 120
PREGNANCY
(also Obstetrics, Ovation).......... 120
PRESCRIPTION 121
PRESCRIPTION
DIRECTIONS 121
PROCRASTINATION 121
PROCTOLOGIST
(also Colon)............................... 121
PROCTOSCOPE........................ 122
PROSIT
(also Atonic, Drinking).............. 122
PROZAC.................................... 122
PSYCHEDELI
(also Food, Nutrition)................ 123
PSYCHIATRIST
(also Paranoia) 123
PSYCHOLOGIST....................... 124
PSYCHOTIC 124
PUBERTY 125
QUADRUPLE BYPASS............... 125
QUININE 125
RABIES 126
RADIOLOGIST
(also X-ray) 126
RECTALGIA............................... 126

RELIGION (also Prayer) 126
REMEDY 127
RESTAURANT
(also Food, Nutrition)................. 128
RETINITIS PIGMENTOSA 129
RETIREMENT 129
ROSACEA.................................... 129
SALIVA 129
SCHIZOPHRENIA 130
SCHOOL..................................... 130
SENILITY 130
SEX.. 131
SEXAGENARIAN
(also Age, Geriatrics, Old) 131
SILICONES
(also Breast Implants) 132
SITZ BATH................................. 132
SKELETON 133
SKIN
(also Dermatologist) 133
SLEEP
(also Insomnia)........................... 133
SLEEPING PILL 134
SMILE... 134
SMOKING
(also Nicotines, Tobacco)........... 135
SNORING 135
SORGHUM (also Dentist) 136
SPEAKING 136
SPECIALIST
(also Med Specialization) 137
SPECIMEN
(also Urinalysis) 138
SPORTS
(also Jocular, Foreplay)............... 138
STOOL
(also Constipate, Laxity) 138
STRESSED................................... 139
SUICIDE...................................... 139
SUNBURN 140
SURGERY.................................... 140
SURGEON................................... 141
TATTOO 141
TEETOTALER............................. 142
TELEVISION 142
TESTICLE 143
TIME... 143
TINNITUS (also Noise) 143

TOASTS....................................... 144
TOBACCO
(also Nicotines, Smoke) 145
TOOTHPASTE 145
TOUPEE...................................... 145
TRANQUILIZERS 146
TRAVEL....................................... 146
TUBERCULOSIS 147
URINAL....................................... 148
URINALYSIS
(also Specimen)........................... 148
UROLOGY
(also Diuretics, Kidney) 148
VALUES 149
VEGETARIAN............................. 149
VETERINARIAN
(also Pets, Polyestrous) 150
VIAGRA 150
VIRUS 150
VITAMIN 151
VOLUNTEER.............................. 151
WAR AND PEACE 152
WARFARIN 152
WEATHER 153
WHISKEY.................................... 153
WINE.. 154
WOMEN 154
WORDS....................................... 155
WORK 156
WRINKLES
(also Botox) 157
WRITING
(also Novelty) 157
X-RAY
(also Radiologist) 158
YAWN 158
YOUTH 158
ZZZZZ... 159

AAAAA
…a club for drinking drivers.
Addendumb: If you drink, don't park. Accidents cause people.

Give them a call and they'll tow you away from the bar and your friends.

If you should need a shoulder to cry on, pull off to the side of the road.

AAADD
Age Activated Attention Deficit Disorder.

It's never too late to have a happy childhood.

On his 85th birthday, George Burns was asked if he had a happy childhood.
He answered, "So far."

ABDOMINAL
…the temple of god, Stomach, in whose worship,
with sacrificial rights, all true men engage.
                              Ambrose Bierce
                              1842-1914

He must have had a magnificent build before his stomach went in for a
career of its own.
                              Margaret Halsey

When I began practice, I was relatively safe in assuming (that abdominal
pain) was appendicitis or green apples. Today it is also highly probable
that the patient is suffering from the fact that his wife of forty years wants
to leave him for the Peace Corps or Richard Burton.
                              Dr. Gunnar Gunderson

Abdicate: to give up all hope of ever having a flat stomach.

Anybody who believes that the way to a man's head is through his stomach
flunked geography.
                              Margaret Halsey

ACNE VULGARIS
…zit happens.

Remember when the teenage drug problem was finding what worked on acne.

Now first he had acne vulgaris,
The kind that was rampant in Paris.
It covered his skin
From forehead to shin.
Now they ask where his hair is.

ACUPUNCTURE
…a jab well done.

The doctor's after-hours advice to patient on the phone:
"Sit on a couple of tacks and call me in the morning."

ADDICT
…one who believes that where there's life, there's dope.

Mainlining: Vein pursuit.

Addiction: a junkie with a gift of gab.

When asked why he ignored the money when robbing the pharmacy,
the addict said, "If I wanted money, I would have robbed a bank."

ADVERTISING
…the art of separating people from their money.

Classified Classics:
For Sale: An antique desk suitable for lady with thick legs and large drawers.
Dog for Sale: Eats anything and is fond of children.
Used Cars: Why go elsewhere to be cheated? Come here first.
Wanted: Man to work in dynamite factory. Must be willing to travel.

The codfish lays ten thousand eggs,
The homely hen lays one.
The codfish never cackles
To tell you what she's done.
And so we scorn the codfish,
While the humble hen we prize,
Which only goes to show you
That it pays to advertise.

Dear Friends:

It is with the saddest heart I pass on the following. Please join me in remembering a great icon — the Pillsbury Doughboy. He died yesterday of a yeast infection and complications from repeated pokes in the belly.

Doughboy was buried in a lightly greased coffin. Dozens of celebrities turned out to pay their respects, including Mrs. Butterworth, Hungry Jack, the California Raisins, Hostess Twinkies, Captain Crunch, Betty Crocker and Drunken Hines.

The gravesite was piled high with flours as longtime friend Aunt Jemima delivered the eulogy describing Doughboy as a man who never knew how much he was kneaded. Doughboy rose quickly in show business, but in his later life was filled with turnovers. He was not considered a very "smart" cookie, wasting much of his dough on half-baked schemes. Despite being a little flaky at times, as a crusty old man he was considered a roll model for millions.

AEROSOLS
…inhalant drugs, which if you are full of and sneeze, can cure someone.

Nasal Spray Salesman:
a guy who goes around sticking his business up other people's noses.

AGING
The seven ages of man:
Spills, drills, thrills, bills, ills, pills, and wills.

Richard Needham

I'm so old bartenders check my pulse instead of my ID.

Louise Bowie

"Safe sex" means not rolling out of bed.

I just took a leaflet out of my mailbox, informing me that I can have sex at 73.
I'm sooo happy, because I live at unit 67.
And it will not be far to walk home afterwards.

My husband will never chase another woman.
He's too fine, he's too decent, he's too old.

Gracie Allen
(when George Burns was only 64)

I get up every morning and dust off my wits
Go pick up the paper and read the O-*bits*.
If my name isn't there I know I'm not dead:
I get a good breakfast and go back to bed.
The reason I know my youth is all spent,
My get-up and go has got-up and went.

AIDS
Senior citizens are the biggest carriers.
Addendumb: Here's proof — Hearing aids, Band-Aids, Rolaids,
Walking aids, Medicaids, Government aids.

When asking the eighty-year-old couple what gave them the reason to
think they might have AIDS, they replied "We read that you can get it
from annual sex."

The doc who was interviewing a new patient and was considering her risk
factors for HIV asked, "Have you had multiple sexual partners in the past?"
    "Oh, no doctor. Only one at a time."

ALCOHOLIC
...someone who drinks more than his own doctor.

A wife didn't know her husband was an alcoholic until the night he came
home sober.

Acute alcoholic: an attractive drunk.

There was a young fellow named Giver
Who drank till he ruined his liver.
It shriveled and shrank
As he sat there and drank,
Leaving an organ the size of a sliver.

N.H.

ALCOHOLICS ANONYMOUS
...a place where you can get drunk without being noticed.

What's the difference between an alcoholic and a drunkard?
Drunkards don't go to meetings.

Jackie Gleason

What happened in my absinthe?
Absence makes the heart grow fonder.

ALLERGY
...a bitch of an itch.

What's the difference between an itch and an allergy?
Several hundred dollars.

Cuticle: a delightful itch.

There was a young belle of old Natchez
Whose garments were always in patchez.
When comment arose
On the state of her clothes,
She drawled, "When ah itchez, ah scratches."
Ogden Nash
1902-1971

ALZHEIMER'S
Of all the things I've lost, I miss my mind the most.
Addendumb: Most people I know have Someheimers.

What is a benefit of having Alzheimer's?
You're always meeting new friends, and you can hide your own Easter eggs.

The woman said her Alzheimer husband had reached the point where
he could not recognize her. On the next visit to the nursing home, she
asked him, "Mohammad, do you know who I am?" Immediately he
answered, "You're my wife." Then he pointed to the nurse's station and
said, "And I've got four more over there."

In recent years, more money has been spent on breast implants and Viagra
than on Alzheimer's disease research, leading one to wonder: by the year
2030, will there be a large number of people wandering around with big
breasts and erections who can't remember what to do with them?

I'm accustomed to my deafness,
To my dentures, I'm resigned,
I can cope with my bifocals,
But-oh dear! I miss my mind.

AMNESIA
I had amnesia once…maybe twice.

Stephen Wright

Never lend money. It gives people amnesia.
Addendumb: Doctors have finally solved this problem.
They simply make patients pay in advance.

ANATOMY
The body is but a pair of pincers set over a bellows and a stew pan
and the whole fixed upon stilts.

Samuel Butler
1835-1902

I have everything now I had twenty years ago — except now it's all lower.

Gypsy Rose Lee

God wisely designed the human body so that we can neither pat our own
backs nor kick ourselves too easily.

Funny bone: It's not a bone and not funny. It's a spot where the ulnar
nerve touches the humerus. Also not funny: Some suffer from osteoporosis
of the funny bone.

Necking: Whoever named it necking was a poor judge of anatomy.

Groucho Marx

Petting: the study of anatomy in braille.

Shin: a device for finding furniture in the dark.

Spine: add up the spinal column and get a disc count.

A washboard stomach: Men want this or a six-pack to replace the keg they
are carrying around.

Where can a man buy a cap for his knee
Or a key for a lock of his hair?
Can your eyes be called an academy
Because there are pupils there?
In the crown of your head what jewels are found?
Who crosses the bridge of your nose?
Could you use in shingling the roof of your mouth
The nails on the end of your toes?
Could the crook in your elbow be sent to jail?

How can you sharpen your shoulder blades?
Could you sit in the shade of the palm of your hand
Or beat on the drum of your ear?
Does the calf of your leg eat the corn on your toe?
Then why grow corn on the ear?

William Dunkle

ANESTHESIA
...an aroma coma.

Anesthesiologist: One who enjoys passing gas.

The doctor passed gas after surgery and laughed, "That must have been about a 6.5 on the rectal scale."

ANGER
...barbed ire that is just one letter short of danger.

One of my problems is that I internalize everything. I can't express anger. I grow a tumor instead.

Woody Allen

Never go to bed mad. Stay up and fight.

Phyllis Diller

Anti-inflammatory Agent: a gentleman who cools a heated discussion.

The only graceful way to accept an insult is to ignore it. If you can't ignore it, top it; if you can't top it; laugh at it; if you can't laugh at it, it's probably deserved.

When three people call you an ass, put on a bridle.

Spanish Proverb

I've had a few arguments with people, but I never carry a grudge. You know why? While you're carrying a grudge, they're out dancing.

Buddy Hackett

For all your days prepare,
And meet them ever alike:
When you are the anvil, bear —
When you are the hammer, strike.

Edwin Markham

ANOREXIA

...the belief that a waist is a terrible thing to mind.
Addendumb: Bulimia is where the pain in gain lays mainly in the drain.

Not much meat on her, but what's there is choice.

Spencer Tracy
(about Katherine Hepburn)

ANTABUSE (Disulfiram)

...the distillation of red ants to produce formic acid.
Addendumb: It was their last drunken crawl.

The ant has made himself illustrious
Through constant industry industrious.
So what?
Would you be calm and placid
If you were full of formic acid?

Ogden Nash

ANTIBIOTICS

The mud of one country is the medicine of another.

Afghanistan Proverb

Chiefly, the mold of a man's fortune is in his own hands.

Francis Bacon
1561-1626

Anti-body: against everyone.

The trouble with being a hypochondriac these days
is that antibiotics have cured all the good diseases.

Caskie Sinnet

APATHY

Pardon my ignorance, but I don't know a thing about this and I don't care.

Scientists announced today that they have discovered a cure for apathy.
However, they claim no one has shown the slightest bit of interest in it.

George Carlin

APHRODISIAC
...a concoction.

Power is the ultimate aphrodisiac.

Henry Kissinger

Rx for romance:
Take the womb of a hare, fry it in a rusted, bronze frying pan, throw in three pounds of rose oil, then make it smooth with good smelling myrrh. Add four drams of fat, one dram of crocodile dung, two drams juice of garlic germander and of bloody flux, and four drams of honey. Drink and get ready for a romantic evening.

Metro Dora
Ancient Greek physician

APOTHECARY
...the physician's accomplice, undertaker's benefactor, and grave's worm provider.

Ambrose Bierce

An apothecary should never be out of spirits.

Richard Brinsly Sheridan
1751-1816

Dead flies cause the ointment of the apothecary to send forth a stinking savour: so doth a little folly him that is in reputation for wisdom and honor.

Ecclesiastes 10:1

Addendumb: Live flies are the worst.

APPENDIX
...An organ that is useless to man but of value to doctors.

Doctor: "You have acute appendicitis."
Female Patient: "I came here to be examined, not admired."

ARTERY
...the gallery of fine art.

For forty-seven days in 1961, the painting "Matisse's Le Bateau (The Boat)" was hanging upside down in the Museum of Modern Art in New York City. Apparently none of the 116,000 visitors seemed to have noticed.

A zealous art student went to a gallery and spent a bewildered hour looking over abstract and cubist works. She was finally attracted to a painting consisting of a black dot on a field of white and framed in brass.

"How much for this?" she asked.

The man answered, "Oh, that's the light switch."

The art of medicine consists of amusing the patient while nature cures the disease.

Voltaire
1694-1778

The artery carries the blood to or from the heart.
I forget which, but the body remembers, and that's the important thing.

ARTHRITIS
...twinges in the hinges caused by pain in the joints.
Addendumb: Stay out of those joints.

For old-timers sake: First we went to a disco party; then we did the twist. This was followed by an ibuprofen party. Then later, a joint replacement party.

After the beautiful young dancer twisted her chronically weak ankle for the third time in as many weeks, the chiropodist said, "I just don't understand what a joint like this is doing in a nice girl like you."

ATONIC
Research suggests that drinking one or two a day is beneficial.

The first glass for myself, the second for my friends,
the third for good humor and the fourth for mine enemies.

Sir William Temple

Those dry martinis did the work for me;
Last night at twelve I felt immense,
Today I feel like thirty cents.
My eyes are bleared and red, my coppers hot,
I'll try to eat, but I cannot.
It is no time for mirth and laughter,
The cold, grey dawn of the morning after.

George Ade

AUTOINTOXICATION
...a wreck just waiting to happen.

A motorist ran over a dog and tried to console its owner.
"I'll be happy to replace your pet."
She replied, "Mister, don't flatter yourself."

Radar spelled backwards is radar; they've got you coming and going.
Bill Leary

Parkinsonism: The feeling you get when someone takes the last parking space.

Sign on highway: Drive carefully. We have two cemeteries and no hospital.
It's not only cars that can be recalled by their makers.

Beneath this slab
John Brown is stowed.
He watched the ads
And not the road.

Ogden Nash

AUTOPSY
...remains to be seen.

Live fast, die young and leave a good-looking corpse.
John Derek
Knock On Any Door

Coroner: The easiest job in the world. What's the worst thing that can happen?
If everything went wrong, maybe you'd get a pulse.
Dennis Miller

BACTERIA
...the backdoor of a cafeteria.

Salmonella is a bacterium that in the human bloodstream can grow into
an adult salmon.
Dave Barry

Support bacteria. It's the only culture some people have.
Addendumb: My sister is so cultured, you could name a yogurt after her.

Before I heard the doctors tell
Of the dangers of a kiss,
I had considered kissing you
The nearest thing to bliss.
But now I know biology
And sit and sigh and moan,
Six million mad bacteria,
And I thought we were alone.

BALDNESS
...follicularly challenged.

An old remedy for baldness is made of alum and persimmon juice.
It doesn't grow hair, but it shrinks your head to fit what hair you have.

If you're after something new, try a drug, a rug or a plug.

If a man is bald in front, he's a thinker. If he's bald in back, he's a lover.
If he's bald in front and back, he thinks he's a lover.

When others kid me about being bald, I simply tell them that the way I
figure it, the good Lord only gave men so many hormones, and if others
want to waste theirs on growing hair, that's up to them.

John Glenn
Astronaut

Balderdash: a rapidly receding hairline.

Two bald-headed men put their heads together,
and they only made an ass of themselves.

I feel so bad for Uncle Ted.
There's not much hair upon his head.
And what is worse, he barely hears —
There's too much hair inside his ears.

Bruce Lansky

BANDAGE
...the age when swing was king.
And it don't mean a thing if it ain't got that swing.

Big Bands: The music is gone, but the malady lingers on.

What do you get when you drop a piano down a mine shaft?
A-flat minor.

The warden threw a party at the county jail,
The prison band was there an' they began to wail.
The brass band was jumpin' an' the joint began to swing.
You should have heard those knocked out jailbirds sing.

Leiber and Stoller, 1957
Jailhouse Rock

BEAUTY
...is in the eye of the beer holder.

W.C. Fields

Laugh and the world laughs with you — cry and you streak your mascara.

Beauty always comes from within — with-in jars, tubes and compacts.

The average girl would rather have beauty than brains,
because the average guy can see better than he can think.

The Circle

The genitals have not undergone the development of the rest of the
human form in the direction of beauty.

Sigmund Freud

"Sig, I hope you're speaking for yourself."

Bathing Beauty: a girl worth wading for.

Somebody once asked me, "Do you like bathing beauties?"
I said, "I don't know, I never bathed one."

Milton Berle

Natural Beauty: It takes at least two hours in front of a mirror.

Pamela Anderson

Addendumb: And a Raving Beauty
is the one who finishes last in a beauty contest.

I once wore a peekaboo blouse. People would peek, then they'd boo.

Phyllis Diller

As a beauty I'm not a great star.
There are others more handsome, by far,
But my face — I don't mind it
Because I'm behind it;
It's the people in front get the jar.

Anthony Euwer

BEER BELLY
...little more than a backup fuel-storage unit.

Give a man a fish and he will eat for a day.
Teach a man to fish and he will sit in a boat and drink beer all day.

Dunlop Disease:
Inflationary disease in which your belly has dunlopped over your belt.
Addendumb: If you're planning to retire, work on your spare now.

Drinking beer doesn't make you fat, it makes you lean
— against bars, tables, chairs, and poles.

BEDPAN
...a type of humor.

Pecan: a hillbilly bedpan.

Bedpandemonium: when all hell breaks loose.

The ultimate indignity is to be given a bedpan by a stranger
who calls you by your first name.

Maggie Kuhn

When visiting someone who's sickly,
Here's a problem that can be tickly —
If they call for a bedpan,
Just react with a dead pan,
Then get out of the room — and quite quickly.

BELLADONNA
...a sight for sore eyes.

In Italian, a beautiful lady,
In English, a deadly poison.
A striking example of the essential identity of the two tongues.

Ambrose Bierce

BERIBERI (lack of Vitamin B1)
On land or sea
One need not be wary.
A well-made *Old-Fashioned*
Prevents beriberi.
Forget your hurry scurry
Downing two will undo scurvy.
And as for rickets,
Why defy them?
When you can simply
Liquefy 'em.

N.H.

BIRTH CONTROL
...multiplication tabled.

Should women have children after thirty-five?
No, thirty-five children is more than enough.

A young woman was calling a record store, but she dialed the wrong number.

When a man answered, she asked: "Do you have 'Eyes of Blue' and
'Love That's Real'?" The perplexed fellow replied, "I don't know, but I've
got a wife and eleven children." The woman asked, "Is that a record?"
He replied, "I don't think so, but it's as close as I want to get."

Mary Zyglowicz

There was an old lady who lived in a shoe.
She didn't have any children —
She knew what to do.

BISEXUAL
...a man who likes girls as well as the next guy.

I can't understand why more people aren't bisexual.
It would double your chances for a date on Saturday night.

Woody Allen

15

BLIND

A blind man comes into a pharmacy and starts knocking things off the shelf with his cane. The manager says, "Can I help you?" He says, "No, thanks, just looking."

People say to the blind "Alex, why not sunglasses?"
I say, "Hey, I don't see deaf people wearing earmuffs."

Alex Valdez
Blind Stand-Up Comedian

I had plenty of pimples when I was a kid. I fell asleep in the library. When I woke up, a blind man was reading my face.

Rodney Dangerfield

BLOOD PRESSURE

The doctor wanted to lower my sodium intake, but I took his advice with a grain of salt.

As for me, except for an occasional heart attack, I feel as young as I ever did.

Robert Benchley

Doctor to blood pressure patient: "I'll make it real easy for you. Just don't eat anything out of a bag."

Plasma: a blud light.

Roses are red,
Violets are blue
Without your lungs
Your blood would be too.

Susan Ott
New England Journal of Medicine

BODY DONATION

...a gift from those who prefer to rest in pieces.

I'm sending my sinuses to Phoenix
My liver to Malibu
My lungs to UCLA
My kidney to Sidney
But my heart is only for you.

N.H.

BODY PIERCING
...a powerful compelling visual statement that says,
"Gee, in today's market, what can I do to make myself less employable?"
Dennis Miller

I think men who have a pierced ear are better prepared for marriage.
They've experienced pain, and bought jewelry.
Rita Rudner

Have you heard of this unbelievable Ad?
Now is your chance to have your ears pierced and get an extra pair to take home, too.

I saw a teenager who had a ring in her nose and eyebrow, and a stud through her tongue. She looked like she had fallen face first into a tackle box.

BOTOX
...wrinkle zapping.

With mirth and laughter, let old wrinkles come.
William Shakespeare
The Merchant of Venice

Botox parties: The doctor brings the syringes, giving new meaning of doing shots at *Happy Hour.*

Due to some doctor's sloppy writing, instead of being taken to Detox, she was taken to Botox. She's still drinking and drugging herself like there's no tomorrow, but she looks fabulous.

BRAIN
I use not only all the brains I have, but all I can borrow.
Woodrow Wilson

It's an apparatus with which we think that we think.
Ambrose Bierce

If the right side of the brain controls the left side of the body, then only left-handed people are in their right minds.

Brains are not a handicap to a girl because a smart girl knows enough to hide them behind a low neckline.

Since I blew my mind, I have been a more open human being.

I have a bone to pick with fate.
Come here and tell me girlie.
Do you think my mind is maturing late,
Or simply rotted early?

BREAST IMPLANTS
They are not only a potential health hazard,
but they violate the truth-in-packaging laws.

Mike Royko

In California you can get breast augmentation surgery on an outpatient basis in about thirty minutes. They call it "Jiffy Boob."

Pamela Anderson confirmed that she has had her breast implants removed. Doctors say she is doing fine and that her old implants are now dating Charlie Sheen.

Conan O'Brien

Busts and bosoms have I known
Of various shapes and sizes,
From grievous disappointments
To jubilant surprises.

Waldo Pierce

BraVo!

BRONCHODILATOR
...horse serum.
Addendumb: It enables a race horse to take several thousand people for a ride at the same time.

Drowning himself in mint juleps after his Kentucky Derby entry broke an ankle, the owner was sad to say, "A horse divided against itself cannot stand."

N.H.

BUCCAL
...something that holds up your pants.

Tokyo commuter Katsuo Katugoru caused havoc on a crowded subway train when his homemade rubber underpants, designed to inflate thirty times their original size in the event of a tidal wave, unexpectedly went off when he reached into his pants.

BULLDOZER
…bovine tranquilizer.

Faith can move mountains, but it is a lot easier with a bulldozer.
Addendumb: That's a lot of bull.

This talk is like a big steer's head
The likeness can be seen
A point right here, another there
And a lot of bull in between.

CANCER
...a smoking cure.

What do you call a person with recurrent lymphoma?
A lymphomaniac.

(Heard at a cancer support group)

I wish I had the voice of Homer
To sing of rectal carcinoma,
This kills a lot more chaps, in fact,
Than were bumped off when Troy was sacked…
I know that cancer often kills,
But so do cars and sleeping pills;
And it can hurt one till one sweats,
So can bad teeth and unpaid debts.
A spot of laughter, I am sure,
Often accelerates one's cure.
So let us patients do our bit
To help the surgeons make us fit.

J.B. Haldane
Cancer's a Funny Thing

CARDIAC ARREST
...getting caught having a card up your sleeve at the casino.
N.H.

Ace Inhibitor: a trump card for one of life's bad deals.

When you get to my age, getting a second opinion is like switching slot machines.

James Walker

My wife and I were in Las Vegas, where she called down for room service.
A half-hour later they sent up a table and a dealer.

Gambling Casino Sign:
If you have a gambling problem — Call 1-800-GAMBLER.
Why not call them and say, "I have an ace and a six.
The leader has a seven. What do I do?"

CATASTROPHE
...top prize for the cat with the most beautiful behind.
Addendumb: The booby prize was a dish of spiked catnip.

Catharsis: a cat coughing up a hairball.

When visitors to your house see a cat's litter box, they always say,
"Oh, have you got a cat?" Just once I want to say, "No, it's for company."

CELEBRITY WORSHIP SYNDROME
...the inability to hitch your wagon to the stars.
                                                    N.H.

The nice thing about being a celebrity is that when you bore people,
they think it's their fault.
                                        Henry Kissinger

Keep your cotton-picking hands off my gin.
                                        Eli Whitney

If life was fair, Elvis would be alive and all the impersonators would be dead.
                                        Johnny Carson

When you shoot for the moon and you come up short, you still end up in
the stars.
                                        Les Brown

I can match bottoms with anyone in Hollywood.
                                        Mia Farrow
"Mia, get too big for your britches and you'll be exposed in the end."

CHIGGER

Here's to the chigger
The bug that's no bigger
Than the point of a pin.
But the bump that it raises
Itches like blazes,
And that's where the rub comes in.

Chigger remedy: apply alcohol and sand. The alcohol puts the chiggers in a frenzy and they all end up throwing rocks at each other.

CHIROPRACTOR

...one who works his fingers to your bones.

Some are proud to be called "slipped disc jockeys."

CHOLESTEROL

...the chemical that ruined meat's reputation.

Confronting a burly butcher at a grocery store one day, my mother requested a piece of beef with no fat and no bone. "Lady," came the reply, "we've been trying to grow them like that for years, but they just fall over."

Cholesterol is poisonous,
So never, never eat it.
Sugar too, may murder you,
There is no way to beat it.
And fatty food may do you in,
Be certain to avoid it.
Some food is rich in vitamins
But processing destroys it.
So let your life be ordered
By each documented fact,
And die of malnutrition
But with arteries intact.

CIRCULATION

A tight girdle can both harm a woman's circulation and increase her circulation.

They told me I had type A blood, but it was a Type O.

Blood vessels: They are made up of the arteries, veins and caterpillars, followed by the corpuscles.

(from student test)

CLAUSTROPHOBIA
...fear of Christmas.

The Magi were truly wise.
Unlike most men, they stopped to ask for directions.

The main reason Santa is so jolly is because he knows where all the bad girls live.

What did the flying reindeer say after eating the magic mushrooms?
"Man, I'm Thor."

What I don't like about Christmas parties is looking for a job the next day.
Phyllis Diller

You moon the wrong person at an office party
and suddenly you're not "professional" any more.
Jeff Foxworthy

The contest was simple. Which department in the hospital could create the best Christmas decorations? While they didn't win first prize, the members of the proctology department did receive high honors with their distinctive sign, "Christmas is a good time to look up old friends."
Pat Ingels

If Christmas is a source of fear
Replacing the usual merry cheer,
Look beyond the holly daze and see
A new year free of auld anxiety.

N.H.

CLOWN
...is like an aspirin, only works twice as fast.
Groucho Marx

Everyone said women love a guy who is funny.
So I dressed up as a clown. I got nowhere.

The arrival of a good clown exercises a more beneficial influence upon the health of a town than twenty asses laden with drugs.

Thomas Sydenham, M.D.
1624-1689

Addendumb: Were those asses pharmacists?

Wouldn't it be great if we could clone a clown?
Remember, a clone is people two.
And we need more Fun-addicts.

And where are the clowns?
Quick, send in the clowns.
Don't bother, they're here.

Steven Sondheim

"Just 'cause you got the monkey off your back doesn't mean the circus has left town."

George Carlin

COCAINE
…the drug to avoid if you don't want to pay through the nose.

It's God's way of saying, "You're making too much money."

Robin Williams

Cocaine isn't habit-forming. I should know. I've been using it for years.

Tallulah Bankhead

I've asked, "What is it about cocaine that makes it so wonderful?" And they say, "It intensifies your personality." But what if you're an asshole?

Bill Cosby

I tried sniffing Coke once. Some say it was snorting.
I quit when the ice stuck in my nose.

Some get a kick from cocaine.
I'm sure that if I took even one sniff
That would bore me terrific'ly too,
Yet I get a kick out of you.

Cole Porter (1934)

He also got his kicks on Route 66.

COCKTAIL PARTY
…where you meet people who drink so much you can't remember their names.

A congressman was once asked about his attitude toward whiskey.
"If you mean the demon drink that poisons the mind, pollutes the body, desecrates family life and inflames sinners, then I'm against it. But if you mean the elixir of Christmas cheer, the shield against winter chill, the taxable potion that puts needed funds into public coffers to comfort crippled children, then I'm for it. This is my position and I will not compromise."

Mark Edw. Lender
and Kirby Martin

COFFEE
...break fluid.

If it weren't for caffeine, some people would have no personality at all.

Latte: Latin for "lotta cals."

Innoculatte: coffee taken intravenously.

Washington Post

Only Irish coffee provides in a single glass all four essential food groups: alcohol, caffeine, sugar, and fat.

Caffeine is my shepherd; I shall not doze.
It maketh me to wake in the lecture hall,
It leadeth me beyond the sleeping masses.
It restoreth my buzz.
It leadeth me in the paths of consciousness for its name sake.
Yea, though I walk through the valley of the shadow of addiction,
I will fear no decaf, for thou art with me.
Thy cream and thy sugar, they comfort me.
Thou preparest a tall latte before me in the presence of fatigue.
Thou anointest my day with pep: my mug runneth over.
Surely richness and taste shall follow me all the days of my life,
And I will dwell in the House of Java forever.

COLD
...a physical ailment that is both positive and negative;
sometimes the eyes have it and sometimes the nose.

William Lyon Phelps

Last week I got a cold, so I took a decongestant that opens the nasal passages. And while they were opened, I caught another cold.

Laser-beam surgery
And test-tube babies,
Bypass techniques
And new shots for rabies.
Medical advances
Are dramatic and bold,
But here I sit
With my common cold.

Mimi Kay
Wall Street Journal

COLD REMEDY
There is only one way to treat a cold and that is with contempt.

William Osler M.D.
1849-1919

If you think you caught a cold, call in a good doctor.
Call in three good doctors and play bridge.

Robert Benchley

Fill mouth with water
Sit on a hot stove and bring close to a boil.
Your cold is gone.

Whiskey is by far the most popular of all remedies that won't cure a cold.

Jerry Vale

Pardon me to appear so bold
In asking how you treat a cold.
"Feed it," they say, "is good advice."
Or, was it, conversely, versa vice?

N.H.

COLON
The three parts of the small intestine are the duodenum, ileum and the odyssey.
Addendumb: Then there is the Sigmoid, or is this a Freudian slip?

Colostomy: when your colon is reduced to a semi-colon.

Intestinal grippe: an illegal wrestling hold.

There was a young man with a hernia
Who said to his doctor, "Gol dernia,
When improving my middle,
Be sure you don't fiddle
With matters that don't concernia."

COLOSSAL
...the large intestine.
Addendumb: Proctologists have assets of colossal proportions.

There's a divinity that shapes our ends, rough-hew them how we will.
William Shakespeare
Hamlet

You think American TV commercials are bad? In Australia there is one
for Rectinol, an ointment "for hemorrhoidal distress." It opens with a
squirming, unhappy string quartet playing Mozart horribly. Then a happy,
beaming quartet playing beautifully as a voice-over says, "Rectinol!
It's music to your rears!"

Prayer of the Large Intestine: O Saint Elena the Rather Plump, I beg your
favor to punish and kill the devils that have taken adverse possession of my
normally rugged digestive system. And , O Thunder Thighs, I have lost
fifteen pounds in the last three days and would be willing to make a
special pilgrimage every year to your shrine in Cancun if I do not gain
this weight back, your Holy Circumference.
Howard Tomb
Wicked Spanish

COMEDIC
...a hospital clown who teams up with your doctor.

When a hospital clown dies, is he at wit's end?
Not if there's a grin reaper to replace him.

God is a comedian playing to an audience too afraid to laugh.
Voltaire

Comic-kazes: the guys whose jokes bombed.

If I get a laugh, I'm a comedian. If I get a small laugh, I'm a humorist. If I get
no laughs, I'm a singer. If my singing gets big laughs, I'm a comedian again.
George Burns

They laughed when I said I was going to be a comedian.
They're not laughing now.

Bob Monkhouse

COMMUNICATION
…evening news where they begin with "Good Evening,"
and then proceed to tell you why it is not.

I have e-mail, a pager, cell phone, car phone, home fax, office fax.
I also have an answering machine, voice mail, video i-pod, blackberry,
web browser, blogger, camera, face book, U-tube, and palm organizer.
If I didn't return your call, I'm experiencing a breakdown.

Phone phooey: I phoned a friend of mine, but got her answering machine
instead. The message said, "Hello, this is you-know-who, and we're not
you-know-where, so at the you-know-when, leave a you-know-what and
we'll…you know!"

The Psychiatric Hotline:
If you are obsessive-compulsive, press one repeatedly.
If you are co-dependent, please ask someone to press *two*.
If you have multiple personalities, press *three, four, five and six*.
If you are paranoid-delusional, we know who you are and what you want.
    Just stay on the line so we can trace your call.
If you are schizophrenic, listen up.
    A little voice will tell you which number to press.
If you are manic-depressive, it doesn't matter which number you press.
    No one cares.

COMPUTER FATIGUE
…when your megabytes become megahertz.
That's 1,000,000 aches.

Computers make it easy to do a lot of things, but most of the things
they make it easier to do, don't need to be done.

Andy Rooney

Am I on Face-Book?
Yes, but I'd rather have my face in a book.

COMPUTER VIRUS
….terminal illness.

Troy Roberts

Ever notice the older we get, the more we're like computers?
We start out with lots of memory and drive, then we become outdated,
and eventually have to get our parts replaced.

COMPUTER DEAF (for those before computers)

Memory was something you lost with age.
A Program was a TV show.
A Curser used profanity.
A Keyboard was on a piano.
A Web was a spider's home.
A Virus was the flu.
A CD was a bank account.
A Hard Drive was a long trip on a road.
A Mouse Pad was where a mouse lived.
And if you had a three and a half inch Floppy
…you just hoped nobody found out.

CONDOM
Using a condom you will learn — no deposit means no return.

Condoms aren't completely safe.
A friend of mine was wearing one and got hit by a bus.
                                        Bob Rubin

Condomnation: a country which bans condoms.

A man goes into a drugstore to buy a pack of condoms. When he pulls out
his wallet to pay, he notes that the bill is thirty-two cents higher than the
price on the box. He asks why and is told that the extra money is for tax.
    "Gee," he muses aloud. "I wondered what held them up."

CONSTIPATION
…to have and to hold.

According to statistics, a man eats a prune every 20 seconds.
I don't know who this fellow is, but I know where to find him.

Cantankerous: one who is constipated and drunk at the same time.

Like my Momma always said,
"Life is like a box of chocolates. You never know what you're going to get."
Tom Hanks
Forrest Gump

COSMETICS
...applied art.

Never use anything that stinks, stings, or stains.
Guide to Miss Piggy's Life

Your forehead is frownless
By botox paralyzed.
Your lips are fuller
By injection collogenized.
Your face lift secured,
Your scalp satirized.
Your flawless complexion
By laser vaporized.
Your thighs are lean
By liposuction minimized.
Your breasts are firm
By implants maximized.
Then why are you surprised
When you're not recognized.

Bina Goldfield in N.Y. Times
Portrait of a Lady

COUGH
...convulsions of the lungs, vellicated by some sharp serosity.
Samuel Johnson
1709-1784

Sign in drugstore: Try our cough syrup. You will never get any better.

A cure for your cough that's precise
Is a gallon of prune juice on ice.
You should really be told
That it won't cure your cold,
But before you cough, you'll think twice.

COUNTER IRRITANT
...a person who should be kept out of the pharmacy,
whereas over-the-counter irritants should be thrown out.

N.H.

Women are more irritable than men,
the reason being that men are more irritating.

CRABS
What's the difference between lice and crabs?
One crawls while the other talks.

Never treat them; because look what they're doing to you.

I had an unusual case of crabs. Most people get that from someone else
who has it already. I got it directly from a crabmeat cocktail.

Ed Bluestone

Florida restaurant sign: Promise her anything, but give her crabs.

Charlie's Shrimp Bucket

Cootie: a good-looking louse.
This used to be the worst thing you could catch from the opposite sex.

Butterflies have wings of gold,
Moths have wings of flame,
Toilet crabs have no wings at all,
But they got there just the same.

CRIME
You can get farther with a kind word and a gun than you can get with a
kind word alone.

Al Capone

Criminals broke into the pharmacy after hours and took all of the Viagra.
Soon apprehended, the police were quick to remark, "The arrest was
simple, for they were all hardened criminals."

A California policeman pulled a car over and told the driver that because
he'd been wearing a seatbelt, he had just won $5000 in a statewide safety
competition. "What are you going to do with the money?" asked the
policeman.
    "Well, I guess I'm going to get a driver's license," he answered.

"Oh, don't listen to him," said the woman in the passenger seat. "He's a smart aleck when he's drunk."

This woke up the guy in the back seat, who took one look at the cop and moaned, "I knew we wouldn't get far in a stolen car."

At that moment there was a knock from the trunk, and a voice said in Spanish, "Are we over the border yet?"

Funny Times

(My Personal Incident):
It was payday night during my basic training course at Ft. Knox, Kentucky. Walking back toward the barracks from the post library, two men stuck a pistol in my stomach and I ended up forking over a month's allowance. When a similar incident happened to Jack Benny, he handled it differently. His crook said, "Your money or your life." After a long pause, the gunman yelled, "Well!" Jack thoughtfully answered, "I'm thinking. I'm thinking."

Answering Machine Message:
There's nobody home now to answer the phone,
So please leave a message when you hear the tone.
But if you're a burglar, we're not gone at all —
We're cleaning our shotguns while screening your call.

Mark Benthall

CRYOTHERAPY

There is a crying for wine in the streets;
all joy is darkened, the mirth of land is gone.

Bible
Isaiah, XXIV, II

Try laughing. Start with a mimicry. Then fake it till you make it. Addendumb: Then laugh so hard that tears run down your leg.

Neurologists have discovered that the reason babies cry right after they are born is that they instinctively understand the magnitude of the national debt they are going to be saddled with.

Richard Lederer

It takes a big man to cry. But it takes a bigger man to laugh at that man.

DANCE THERAPY

I learned dancing from Arthur Murray.
Later I found out it was more fun with a girl.

Passion is for people who can't polka.

Old German Proverb

Belly dancing is the only profession where the beginner starts in the middle.

My father originated the limbo dance — trying to get into a pay toilet.

Slappy White

Ballet demands discipline, skill, athleticism, perseverance and courage.
And that's just to get into the tights.

Rumba is a dance where the front of you goes along nice and smooth like
a Cadillac and the back of you makes like a jeep.

Bob Hope

I grew up with fourteen in our family. That's how I learned to dance —
waiting to get into the bathroom.

You're asking me to slam dance? Young lady, you're looking at someone
who's done the Cakewalk, the Dipsy Doodle, the Big Apple, the
Charleston, the Bunny Hop, the Shag, the Continental, the Carioca,
the Stomp, the Lindy Hop, the Twist, and the Mashed Potato.
But a slam dance at my age could easily turn into a break dance!

DATING
A man chases a woman until she catches him.

American Proverb

"I want a good girl…and I want her bad."

Don McGill

Addendumb: Just like the one that married dear old Dad.

An archaeologist is the best husband any woman can have.
The older she gets, the more interested he is in her.

Agatha Christie

Want ad: Young Republican woman would like to marry young Democrat.
Object? Third party.

I once dated a famous Aussie rugby player who treated me just like a
football: made a pass, played footsie, then dropped me as soon as he scored.

Kathy Lette

Our days will be so ecstatic,
Our nights will be so exotic.
For I'm a neurotic erratic
And you're an erratic erotic.

E.Y. Harburg

DEATH
...esprit de corpse.

You cannot die laughing, but you could end up dead serious.

A natural death is where you die by yourself without the aid of a doctor.

Mark Twain

For three days after death, hair and fingernails continue to grow,
but phone calls taper off.

Johnny Carson

If Shaw and Einstein couldn't beat death, what chance have I got?
Practically none.

Mel Brooks

I asked an old gentleman what he thought about euthanasia and he
replied, "I'm not as concerned about those youth as I am with the youth
in this country."

He was a cautious man.
He never romped or even played,
He never smoked, he never drank,
Or even kissed a maid.
And when he up and passed away,
Insurance was denied,
For since he hadn't ever lived,
They claimed he never died.

DENTIST
...one who always looks down in the mouth.

When your jaw is swollen, it's hard to transcend dental medication.

When a youngster was quizzed on how many teeth he had, he replied,
"I have eight canines, eight cuspids, two molars and eight cuspidors."

Dentist's tombstone: Stranger! Approach this spot with gravity.
John Brown is filling his last cavity.

The Dentist's favorite hymn: "Crown Him With Many Crowns."

Hygienist, in your dental chair
I sit without a single care,
Except when tickled by your hair.
I know that when you grab the drills
I need not fear the pain that kills.
You merely make my molars clean
With pumice doped with wintergreen.
So I lean back in calm reflection,
With close-up views of your complexion,
And taste the flavor of your thumbs
While you massage my flabby gums.
To me, no woman can be smarter
Then she who scales away my tartar,
And none more fitted for my bride
Then one who knows me from inside.
At least as far as she has gotten
She sees how much of me is rotten.

Earnest A. Hooton
Ode to a Dental Hygienist

DEPRESSION
...merely anger without enthusiasm.

I had to get rid of my therapist. She wasted a lot of time talking.
So I said, "Excuse me, but can we go directly to the medication?"
Maura Kennedy

Bi-Polar: able to grin and bear it.

I was once thrown out of the hospital for depressing other patients.

Seasonal Affective Disorder (SAD):
A little madness in the Spring
Is wholesome, even for the King.

Emily Dickinson

DERMATOLOGISTS
...doctors who start from scratch before making rash judgments.

If it's dry, make it wet.
If it's wet, make it dry.
Your patients don't get well,
But then, they don't die.

John V. Alcott
World Medical News

DIABETES
Give it an inch and it will take a foot.

The police found a fellow lying in the middle of the road, with a bracelet on his wrist and writing on it. "If you find me unconscious, do not give me insulin. I am drunk."

A veterinarian informed a lady that her dog had diabetes.
"How can that be? No one else in our family has had it."

DIAGNOSE
...that part of the body best treated by a plastic surgeon.

My Dad said I was the cutest baby he'd ever seen, except that I had no nose. Then Mom told him he was holding me upside down and backwards.

Rhinoplasty:
The technical term for the nose job is rhinoplasty. Rhino? I mean, do we really need to insult the person at this particular moment in their life? They know they have a big nose, that's why their coming in.

Jerry Steinfield

The Nose:
A bouquet of noses,
We didn't say roses,
Though roses are beautiful and sweet.
Tis the nose that tells us,
Enchants us, compels us
To scents good enough to eat.

DIAGNOSIS
Notice in doctor's waiting room:
To avoid delay, please have all of your symptoms ready.

Woman to doctor: "Before I accept your diagnosis,
I'd like to consult another patient."

Kaz
Modern Medicine

The joy of medicine is the challenge of making a solid diagnosis,
the delight in besting (if only momentarily) an intern or resident,
the satisfaction (if rare) of actually helping someone, the sheer
cantankerousness of being able to tell the bureaucracy to "stuff it."

Dr. Michael J. Halberstam

DIAGNOSTIC
...a funeral of someone who's not sure of his place in the hereafter.

Diagnostician: One finger in the throat and one in the rectum makes a
good diagnostician.

William Osler, M.D.

DIARRHEA
...at loose ends.

It may be hereditary if it runs in your genes.

Listen, my children, and you shall hear
The midnight ride of diarrhea.
Off with the covers, and on to the floor,
A fifty-foot dash to the bathroom door.
"Hasten, Jason, bring the basin."
Plip-plop! "Too late. Bring the mop."

DIET
...comes from the verb, to die.

Art Buchwald

Addendumb: Don't diet, live it.

I told my doctor I get very tired when I go on a diet, so he gave me pep
pills. Know what happened? I ate faster.

Joe E. Lewis

I am lactose intolerant, but I am not opposed to others drinking milk in
moderation.

The two best sellers in any bookstore are the cookbooks and the diet books.
The one tells you how to prepare the food and the other how not to eat any of it.
Andy Rooney

DIETER
...one who starves to death to live a little longer.

My wife is a light eater. As soon as it's light, she starts to eat.
Henny Youngman
Addendumb: Just another refrigeraider.

Vegetables are a must on a diet.
I like carrot cake, zucchini bread and pumpkin pie.

I had to go to the doctors last week. He told me to take all my clothes off.
Then he said, "You'll have to diet." I said, "What color?"
Ken Dodd

A lot of people can't count calories and have the figures to prove it.

Dieter's prayer:
Lord, grant me the strength that I may not fall
Into the clutches of cholesterol.
At polysaturates I'll never mutter,
For the road to hell is paved with butter.
And cake is cursed and cream is awful,
And Satan is hiding in every waffle.
Teach me the evils of hollandaise,
Of pasta and gobs of mayonnaise.
And crisp fried chicken from the South.
Lord, if you love me, shut my mouth.
Dr. Steven A. Pickert

DIGITALIS
...an early form of arithmetic for counting up to twenty.

I once dated a guy who was so dumb he could not count to twenty-one
unless he was naked.
Joan Rivers

DISEASE
...the tax on pleasures.
John Ray (1695)

Illusive: putting off seeing the doctor.

First the doctor told me the good news:
I was going to have a disease named after me.

Steve Martin

Herpes: Half of herpes is her.
And the difference between love and herpes is that herpes lasts forever.

Hereditary diseases: Always bill these to the parents.

Dreaded Furniture Disease (DFD): when your chest is falling into your drawers.

Gout: It's a very singular disease — it seems as if the stomach fell down into the feet.

Sydney Smith

Ulcers: I don't have ulcers; I give them.

Harry Cohn

Doctors say that cheerful people resist disease better than gloomy people. In other words, it's the surly bird who catches the germ.

Physicians of the utmost fame
Were called at once, but when they came,
They answered as they took their fees,
There is no cure for this disease.

Hilaire Belloc
Henry King (1896)

DISEASES
The rabbit's dreary eyes grow dreamier
As he quietly gives you tularemia.
The parrot closes his hooked proboscis
And laughs while handling you psittacosis.
In every swamp or wooded area
Mosquito witches brew malaria.
We risk at every jolly picnic
Spotted fever from a tic nick.
People perish of bubonic.
To rats, it's better than a tonic.
The hog converted into pork
Puts trichinosis on your fork.

The dog today that guards your babies
Tomorrow turns and gives them rabies.
The baby, once all milk and spittle,
Grows to a Hitler, and boy, can he hittle!
That's our planet, and we're stuck with it.
I wish its inheritors the best of luck with it.

Ogden Nash
"A Bulletin Has Just Come In"

DIURETICS
Patient to doctor: "I thought those diuretics were fantastic
until I discovered it was only a leak in the water bed."

"Do I have enough laxatives?" a lady asks at the pharmacy counter.
"You have twenty tablets," I said.
"But are you also drinking enough water to help your condition?"
She answered, "Oh, yes. I'm taking a water pill."

DOCTOR
...one who suffers from good health.

Heal thyself?
Does a doctor doctor a doctor according to the doctored doctors' doctrine
or doctoring, or does the doctor doing the doctoring doctor the other
doctor according to his own doctoring doctrine?

The best doctors in the world are Doctor Diet, Doctor Quiet, and Doctor
Merryman.

Johnathan Swift
1667-1745

Doctors are busy playing God when so few of us have the qualifications.
And besides, the job is taken.

Bernie S. Siegel, M.D.

Doctor to patient:
"You've got to slow down or you're in for a serious breakdown or a heart attack."
(One month later)
Doctor: "How are you?"
"Well, I took your advice and slowed down. Now I lost my job."
Doctor: "Don't worry. I know a good psychiatrist."

Unto our doctors let us drink,
Who cure our chills and ills,
No matter what we really think
About their pills and bills.

DOCTOR'S LIFE
Look up noses
Look down throats
Look up nostrums
Jot down notes
Look up rectums
Look down ears
Look up patients
In arrears.
Pull down covers
Pull up gowns...
Life is full of
Ups and downs.

                                        Richard Armour

It's impossible to get doctors on the phone. I've tried. Every so often I call
my own office just to see, and I can't get me. The best I can do is to leave a
message, and even then it takes me two or three days to get back to myself.
                                        Mark DePaolis, M.D.

DOCTOR ORDERS
No more wine and women, but you can sing all you want.

My husband wasn't listening when the doctor asked for "a urine, stool and
semen sample"...so I just told him they wanted his shorts.

"Your tests are back, don't come any closer!"

My doctor gave me six months to live, but when I couldn't pay the bill,
he gave me six months more.
                                        Walter Matthau

Doctor to hospital patient: "Well, it looks like you're not going to be with
us much longer."
Patient: "Could you be a bit more specific?"

Doctor to patient: Let me put it this way — the softness of your muscles is
exceeded only by the hardness of your arteries.

Give me a doctor, partridge plump,
Short in the leg and broad in the rump,
An endomorph with gentle hands,
Who'll never make absurd demands
That I abandon all my vices,
Nor pull a long face in a crisis,
But with a twinkle in his eye
Will tell me that I have to die.

W.H. Auden

DOCTOR TYPES

Remember, half the doctors in the country graduated in the bottom half of their class.

Al McGuire

DO — Doctor only
Sport — Jock Doc
OB — Fat Doc
ER — Doc in a box
Duo — Paradox
DOA — Late Doc

An elderly doctor was asked why he retired.
"For reasons of health," he replied. "My patients were getting sick of me."

Some doctors I have known: Drs. Cholera, Gass, Hogg, Lucky, Shybut, Uritis, Wiwi, and Sing Song Sung M.D.

DOPAMINE

Don't confuse this with the dope you're dating.

They are a perfect pair. She's a hypochondriac and he's a pill.

Nick and Mary had been dating for many years. Each night after she closed her shop, Mary would go to Nick's place, cook their dinner, wash up and return to her home. One evening after this had gone on for years, she said , "Nick, it's about time we got married." "Oh, Mary," Nick sighed, "Yes, but who would have us?"

DRINKING

Sign in bar: We do not serve women. You must bring your own.

When a girl says she never drinks anything stronger than pop,
maybe you'd better check and see what Pop drinks.

If all be true as we do think,
There are five reasons why we drink:
Good wine, a friend, or being dry,
Or, but we should be, by and by —
Or any other reason why.

Henry Aldrich

Candy is dandy
But liquor is quicker.

Ogden Nash
Reflections on Icebreaking

Addendumb: Today, ornery oracle Ogden Nash would say:
If candy is dandy
And liquor quicker,
Is hash a smash?
No, No, pot is not.

DRUNKARDS
What the sober man thinks, the drunkard tells.

French Proverb

To them a brouhaha is a happy drunk and a problem drinker
is one who never buys.
Addendumb: So let's all go on an Alco-Holiday.

Always do sober what you said you'd do drunk.
That will teach you to keep your mouth shut.

Ernest Hemingway

Stay home when you are drunk.

Euripides, c.484-406 BC
Greek Playwright

"Starkle, starkle, little twink,
Who the deuce you are I tink.
I'm not under the affluence of incohol
As some of you tinkle peep I am.
Why, I'm not half as thunk as you might drink.
But I feel so foolish, I don't know who is me,
And the drunker I stand here, the longer I get. Oh me!"

DRUG ABUSE

Alcohol, pot, tobacco and other drugs do away with half of mankind, but without these, the other half would die.

Those Baby Boomers who used to take acid, now take antacid.

Drug legalization: a cop-out.

Illegal drug: one administered to a sick bird.
Addendumb: Some sick birds are better tweated by quack doctors.

DRUG BUST

...an unexpected Narc at the door.

Drug Dealer: A hero who ends up kissing the heroin goodbye.
N.H.

To criminal suspect: "Do you take drugs?"
"Oh, no man, with my bread, I can now afford them!"

DRUG COMBINATIONS

Never take a laxative and sleeping pill on the same night.

Prozac and Ginkgo: They make you feel good about remembering yourself.

When Viagra, Prozac and Ex-Lax are taken together, these magnify the effects of each other. The result is that you end up both coming and going at the same time. But you couldn't care less.

DRUG NAMES

You say Levoxin and I say Lanoxin.
You say Ciloxin and I say Cibroxin.
Levoxine, Lanoxin, Ciloxin, Cibroxin.
Let's call the whole thing off.

Doug Bennett, R.Ph.

DRUG NAMES (of mistaken identity)

AMBIENCE
ASCENDIN
ANTIDOPE
BAKLOFIN
CONCERTAME
BELLIGO
BORDELLOT
CLOPIDOGRUEL
CELEBREW
DAMNITAL
ENDABUSE
FATATOMY
FATASSNIL
FINASTEROID
FLIPITOR
FORDMOTOROL
FROLIC ACID
GISMO
GLO-LYTELY
GORILLACILLIN
HAFASPRIN
INDERAM INSERTS
LESCOOL
NOTSOCOL XL
LIVIT
LODINER
EMPTYNESTROGEN
ENTERFERNO

WYTENSION
LOVEKNOX
NOTOX
LUNITY
LUNESTAR
MORBID
MORTALIZE
MUSETAB
NOASITAL
NOCOMPRAR
OXYGODONE
ORAPRONOBIS
PRIMADONNA
PHAZEME
PHENOBARBIDOLLS
PROZAP
ROPONAROLL
SADALOT
SEXCEED
SINNOMOR
SUFFRIN
TALWIND
THREEBLINDMYCIN
TRYLAFIN
TUMORBID
SUPERSPERMAN
VIAGRIN
WOEBEGON

DRUG SALES REPRESENTATIVES

On their advice to doctors: "If you don't know what drug to order, always order the drug on your pen."

Rip Pfeiffer, M.D.

Adenoid: bothered by drug representatives.

Those drugs thou hast, and their adoption tried,
Grapple them to thy soul with hoops of steel;
But do not dull thy palm with entertainment
Of each new-hatch'd, unfledged remedy.

William Shakespeare
Hamlet

DRUGSTORE
The brewery is the best drugstore.

German Proverb

Customer at drug counter: "Sorry, I don't know the brand name, but I can hum a few bars of the commercial."

An older patient approached me in my pharmacy with a very irritating wart on her finger. She asked what I would recommend for the wart. After looking at the wart, I told her the best I could offer was a "doctor's visit." A short time later, she returned to my counter and said, "Excuse me, sir, could you kindly tell me where the 'Doctor's Visit' is found?"

Jeff Plunkett, R.Ph

Have you heard about the idiot who put cyanide in the Tylenol?
Well, now there's a jerk who is putting Crazy Glue in our Preparation H.

A grandfather was trying to explain to his grandson what it is like working behind the drugstore's soda fountain years ago. "We made our own Cokes back then" he told him. "We placed a little Coke syrup in a glass, added ice and mixed the whole works from a soda water faucet."

"Gosh Gramps, I had no idea you were around before bottles and cans."

Sign in N.Y. drugstore: We dispense with accuracy.

Sign in Dallas: Observe National Pharmacy Week — Get Sick.

At drugstore counter:
"I'm looking for an athletic supporter."
"What kind, sir?"
"I don't know, what do you have?"
"Well, it all depends on how much you want to put into it."

DRUG TESTING
...urine trouble.

Why is there such controversy about drug testing? I know plenty of guys who'd be willing to test any drug they can come up with.

George Carlin

The boxing decree had a familiar sting,
Drug tests for all who go in the ring.
Those who defied heard the shout,
"It's either urine, or your out!"

N.H.

DYING
Who you going to call? Ghostbusters?
Addendumb: That's like whistling in the dark. If it's during the week,
I would call a good doctor.

I'm not afraid of dying. I just don't want to be around when it happens.
Woody Allen

Dying is easy. Comedy is hard.
Edmund Kean
1833, on deathbed

Dilate: do this and you have a good chance to lead a better life.

Barium: what you do when CPR fails.

News headline headache: The doctor felt the man's purse and said there
was no hope.

Humor keeps the elderly rolling along, singing song. When you laugh,
it's an involuntary explosion of the lungs. The lungs need to replenish
themselves with oxygen. So you laugh, you breathe, the blood runs, and
everything is circulating. If you don't laugh, you'll die.
Mel Brooks

Cremation: for those who think outside the box and want to make an ash
of themselves.

We're all cremated equal.
Goodman Ace

Last Words: This is a sharp medicine, but it is a sure cure for all diseases.
Sir Walter Raleigh
At Execution, 1618

Death has got something to be said for it:
There's no need to get out of the bed for it;
Wherever you may be,
They bring it to you free.
Kingsley Amis
Delivery Guaranteed

EGOTIST
...a person of low taste, more interested in himself than in me.
Ambrose Bierce

The nicest thing about an egotist is that he never goes around talking about other people.

ELECTROCARDIOGRAM
...ticker tape.

As for me, except for an occasional heart attack, I feel as young as I ever did.
                                                                    Robert Benchley

How can you increase the heart rate of your 50-year old husband?
Tell him you're pregnant.
                                                                    P.D. Witte

EMOTION
...a prostrating disease caused by a determination of the heart to the head.
It is sometimes accompanied by a copious discharge of hydrated chloride of sodium from the eyes.
                                                                    Ambrose Bierce

A good rule for going through life is to keep the heart a little softer than the head.
                                                                    Changing Times

Mixed emotions: to see your mother-in-law go over the cliff in your brand new Cadillac.

When we were young, you made me blush,
Go hot and cold, and turn to mush.
I still feel all these things, it's true —
But is it menopause, or you?
                                                                    Susan Anderson

ENEMA
...not a friend.

As a patient, never be your own worst enema.

On the Mike Douglas Show, Don Rickles was singing the praises of a Danny Thomas-produced program entitled "Zero Man." In his enthusiasm for the program, Rickles said, "I wouldn't be a bit surprised if Danny Thomas got an 'Enema Award' for this one."

ENVIRONMENT

I can remember the time when the air was clean and sex was dirty.
George Burns

We've got to pause and ask ourselves: How much clean air do we need?
Lee Iacocca
"Lee, is all the talk of Global Warming just a bunch of hot air?"

Bumper sticker: Life without bears would be unbearable.

What do grizzly bears call mountain bikers? "Meals On Wheels."
Addendumb: And they call joggers "Fast Food."

At the supermarket check-out a bagger asks, "Sir, would you like paper
or plastic?" "Makes no difference, I'm bi-sacksual."

EPILEPSY

...the survival of the fit.

Sign below Hong Kong dress shop: Ladies — Have Fits Upstairs.

One lady was laughing real hard at my jokes.
Then I realized she was having a seizure.

What should you do if you find your dog having a fit in your bathtub?
Throw in your laundry and two cups of Tide.

EPITAPH

...a statement that often lies above about the one that lies below.

In a local cemetery: In memory of my father, gone to join his appendix,
his tonsils, his olfactory nerve, an eardrum, and a leg prematurely removed
by an intern who needed the experience.

Epitaph of Prime Minister Joe Lyons of Tasmania:
Where-ever you may be
O let your wind go free
'Cos holding it caused the death of me.

Here lies the body of Mary Jane Abbott
She burst while drinking an alka tablet
Called from this world to her heavenly rest
She should have waited till it effervesced.

ERECTION
...the stiff of life, the staff of laugh, and often vice versa.

An erection is chiefly caused by scuraum, eryngoes, cresses, parsnips, artichokes, turnips, asparagus, candied ginger, acorns bruised to powder and drunk in muscadel, scallion, and sea shell fish.

Attributed to Aristotle (1684)

Bruised acorns and drunk? It's all Greek to me.

ERECTILE DYSFUNCTION
...the result of faulty flooring.

I bought a product for erectile dysfunction and the box said "Cialis."
I'm still looking for her.

ETHNOBOTANY
...back to our roots.

An ethnobotanist is a born-again plant worshipper.

I take geranium, dandelion, passion flower, and hibiscus.
I feel great and when I pee, I experience the fresh scent of potpourri.

EXERCISE
I like long walks, especially when they're taken by people who annoy me.
Fred Allen

The only reason I would take up jogging is so that I could hear heavy breathing again.
Erma Bombeck

Exercise is human; not to is divine.
Robert Orben

My grandmother started walking five miles a day when she was sixty.
She's ninety-five now, and we don't know where the hell she is.
Ellen DeGeneres

Sign on a farmer's fence: Walkers are allowed to cross the field for free, but remember — the bull charges.
Addendumb: Mugwumps place their mug on one side of the fence and their wumps on the other.

Sleepwalking: a good way to get your rest and your exercise at the same time.

Ironic twist: While men are pumping iron, women are popping Fem-Iron.

Company Notice: We have no physical fitness program. Everyone gets enough exercise by jumping to conclusions, flying off the handle, running down their friends, carrying things too far, dodging issues, passing the buck, and pushing their luck.

When teaching a class on reducing the risk of cardiovascular disease to a group of men, one asked me if sex could be considered an aerobic exercise. I said it was if he could keep it up for 40 minutes three – six times per week.

Mary Carter

In the dim and distant past,
When life's tempo wasn't fast,
Grandma used to rock and knit,
Crochet, tat, and babysit.
Grandma is now at the gym,
Exercising to keep slim.
Now she's golfing with the bunch,
Taking clients out to lunch.
She's going north to ski and curl,
And all her days are in a whirl,
Nothing seems to stop or block her,
Now that Grandma's off her rocker.

EYESIGHT
The eyes are windows on the soul.

Some things have to be believed to be seen.

Ralph Hodgson

My eyes are so bad I can't read menus anymore. I have to order from the pictures on the menu. One time I ordered a bar stool. Then a drunk told me I had psoriasis.

More than 50% of Americans wear glasses,
which gives you some idea of how important the ears are.

My grandmother is over 80 and still doesn't need glasses.
Drinks right out of the bottle.

Henny Youngman

Cauterize: visual contact.

Eyedropper: A clumsy ophthalmologist.

In the 1940s, when Pope John XXIII was still an archbishop and the papal nuncio, or ambassador, in Paris, he was at an elegant dinner party, seated across from a woman wearing a low-cut dress that exposed a good deal of cleavage. Someone turned to him and said, "Your excellency, what a scandal! Aren't you embarrassed that everyone is looking at that woman?" And he said, "Oh no, everyone is looking at me, to see if I'm looking at that woman."

Rev. James Martin S.J.
Between Heaven and Mirth

In Dublin, Mick confided to Mike that he had a problem. "I keep seeing leprechauns, morning, noon and night. It's driving me crazy." Mike asked, "Are you seeing a psychiatrist?" He answered, "No, only leprechauns."

I gaze into her shining eyes
With joy my soul transcends
And yet — I wonder, is it love
Or shiny contact lens?

FAMILIARITY
Happiness is when you have a large, loving, caring, close-nit family in another city.

George Burns

Three of us slept in one bed. When it got cold, Mom threw on another brother. We couldn't afford a watchdog. When we heard a noise at night we'd bark ourselves.

They say when you die there's a light at the end of the tunnel. When my father dies, he'll see the light, make his way toward it, and then flip it off to save electricity.

Harland Williams

One would be in less danger
From the wiles of a stranger
If one's own kin and kith
Were more fun to be with.

Ogden Nash
Family Court

FASHION

…something that goes in one year and out the other.

I know my sister loves me because she gives me all her old clothes and has to go out and buy new ones.

Lauren
Age 4

Clothes don't make the man, but they can break a husband.

Every time a woman leaves off something she looks better, but every time a man leaves off something he looks worse.

Will Rogers

Adam wore the plants in his family and he always wondered how many fig leaves Eve tried on before she said, "I'll take this one."

I know this dress was a bargain because I overheard the clerk in the store say that I got it for a ridiculous figure.

Minnie Pearl

What is Victoria's secret? The secret is that nobody older than 30 can fit into their stuff.

When Shakespeare wrote that there's a divinity that shapes our ends, women didn't wear slacks.

Scotch, anyone?
Is there anything worn under the kilt?
No, it's all in perfect working order.

Spike Milligan

There was a young lady named Jeanie,
Who wore an outrageous bikini,
Two wisps light as air, One here and one there,
With nothing but Jeanie betweenie.

Alan Banks

FATIGUE

The best thing to take when you're run down is the license number of the car that hit you.

Today my heart beat over 103,000 times.
My blood traveled 186,000 miles.
I breathed over 23,000 times.
I inhaled 438 cubic feet of air.
I spoke 4,800 words.
I moved 750 major muscles.
I exercised 7,000,000 brain cells.
No wonder I'm tired.

FEVER
Some doctors are grateful for small fevers.

Fervor: Fever with a purpose.

Spring fever: When the iron in your blood turns to lead in your butt.

Fever remedy: Put the person with a fever in bed with the person with the chills.

Once Antigonus was told that his son, Demetrius, was ill and went to see him. At the door he met some young beauty. Going in, he sat down by the bed and took his son's pulse. "The fever," said Demetrius, "has just left me."
　　"Oh, yes," replied the father. "I met it going out the door."

Plutarch
(c.46-120 AD)

FIRST AID
(from 4th graders): For asphyxiation, apply artificial respiration until patient is dead.

What if a man is bleeding from a wound to the head? Put a tourniquet around his neck.

When would you call for an emetic? Only when you need an ambulance driver.

To stop nosebleed, stand on your head til your heart stops bleeding.

(from adults): No sooner did she leave the first aid course when she was confronted with an emergency.
　　"I saw this accident where a pedestrian was hit by a car. His arm was broken, and his face was covered with blood."
　　"So what did you do?" her friends asked.
　　"Thanks to the first aid course, I knew exactly what to do. I sat down on the curb and put my head between my knees to keep from fainting."

FLABBERGASTED
...the shock of how much weight people say you've accumulated.

N.H.

A word to the wide is sufficient.

Never hold in a laugh. It goes right to the stomach and gives you gas.

FLATULENCE
...a way to unwind.

May the wind be always at your back, unless it's coming from you personally.

Irish Proverb

Fart? No. It's more refined to say "break wind."

Don Marquis

Addendumb: But some don't break it, they "shatter" it.

My prize question: To discover some drug wholesome and not disagreeable, to be mixed with our common food, or sauces, that shall render the natural discharges of wind from our bodies, not only inoffensive, but agreeable as perfumes.

Benjamin Franklin
*Letter to the Royal Academy
of Brusselles, 1781*

If you jog in a jogging suit, lounge in lounging pajamas and smoke in a smoking jacket, why would anyone go near you when you wear a windbreaker?

During a state visit to Great Britain, President Ronald Reagan purportedly went horseback riding with Queen Elizabeth. At one point, one of the horses passed gas quite loudly. The queen apologized, "There are some things even royalty can't control." Reagan replied, "I'm glad you told me, or I would have thought it was the horse."

Readers Digest

As we take on years, we get older and bolder,
Our urges get warmer...control gets much colder!
We no longer hear the sweet music *delectum,*
The symphonic discharge that sings from our rectum.
We know what's occurring and think we are sneaking,
But others around us know well that we're leaking!
When, as guests, we are rising and slowly departing,
The host turns his nose, as we start in to Farting.

I think we should change all the rules of decorum,
By assembling a National Flatulence Forum
To redefine etiquette, in the manner of Sartre,
And soon we will all be admiring the Fartre.

Joel Berman M.D.

FLEAS
One of the best things for fleas is to find them a nice dog.

So naturalists observe, a flea
Hath smaller fleas that on him prey;
And these have smaller still to bite 'em
And so proceed ad infinitum.
Thus every poet, in his kind,
Is bit by him that comes behind.

Jonathan Swift
1667-1745

FLU
If everyone else has a flu shot, you don't need one.

Whiskey may not cure the flu, but it fails more agreeably than most things.

If you're serious about your flu, ask us to go "up yours."

Ad
Whistle Chimney Sweeps

A bunch of germs were hitting it up
In a bronchial saloon.
Two bugs on the edge of the larynx
Were jazzing a hay-feverish tune.
While back of the teeth in a solo game
Sat dangerous Dan Kerchoo.
And watching his pulse was the queen of the waltz,
The lady that's known as Flu.

Cal Beacock

FOOD
I'm on a seafood diet. I see food, I eat it.

Dolly Partin

Listeners in Lafayette, Indiana were shook up when the local station ran two commercials back-to-back, with this unappetizing result: "What are you going to get from Burger Chef? What are you going to get today? …pimples, blackheads, and acne are problems that plague teenagers everywhere."

All mushrooms are edible, but some only once.

Croatian Proverb

Take chopstick and place it between the base of your thumb and your hand, extending outward between your middle and ring fingers. Grasp the other chopstick with the tips of your thumb and index finger. Now, holding the two sticks parallel, raise them over your head and signal to the waiter that you would like him to please bring you a fork.

Dave Barry

The best anti-aging cream is ice cream.
What other food makes you feel like you're 8 years old again?

Chitlins? That's pig intestines! That includes the lower tract. Ain't no food down in that area. Chitlins — I think somebody misspelled that word.

Bill Cosby

Methuselah ate what was on his plate,
Not as people do now.
He never took a calorie count,
He ate because it was chow.
He cheerfully chewed his food
Unmindful of troubles or fears,
Lest his health might be hurt
By some fancy dessert.
And he lived over nine hundred years.

FOOL
There is a foolish corner in the brain of the wisest man.

Aristotle

Make it foolproof and somebody will make a better fool.

There's no fool like an old fool,
but some teenagers can offer some pretty stiff competition.

A clever, ugly man every now and then is successful with the ladies,
but a handsome fool is irresistible.

William Makepeace Thackeray

A fool and his money are "some party."
Addendumb: How did he get the money in the first place?

I sometimes wonder if the manufacturers of foolproof items keep a fool or two on their payrolls to test things.

Alan Coren

Joe came to work looking sheepish and embarrassed. His friend Jim finally pried the problem out of him. Billy explained, "I received a party invitation last night, and it plainly said, "Black Tie Only." But when I got there, everyone else was wearing clothes."

FOOT AND MOUTH DISEASE
A closed mouth gathers no feet.

It is better to keep your mouth shut and appear stupid than to open it and remove all doubt.

Mark Twain

Never put both feet in your mouth at the same time.
Because then you won't have a leg to stand on.

FOREPLAY
...an obsession of amateur golfers.

Give me golf clubs, fresh air and a beautiful partner, and you can keep the clubs and the fresh air.

Jack Benny

Cialis saved my marriage, but now I never get to golf.

Danny Cross

My golf is improving. Yesterday I hit the ball in one.

Sign on golf course: Any persons (except players) caught collecting golf balls on this course will be prosecuted and have their balls removed.

Sportscaster: "Here we are on the fifteenth green where Billy Casper is getting to putt... Billy, usually an excellent putter, seems to be having difficulty with his long putts. However, he has no trouble dropping his shorts."

The rules describe The Game in terms quite sparse:
"To Stroke the Ball with Clubs, within the Rules,
From Tee to Hole." That's it. Sounds like a farce
Engaged in by communities of fools.

Scottish shepherds started this while bored
With tending to their flocks of goats and sheep.
They took up sticks, then swung at stones and scored
Wherever they went in, six inches deep.

Since then, we've fallen to The Games full thrall.
We even took a Titleist to the Moon.
One small step for man, one big for Ball —
No wonder prophets say our doom is soon.

But if you're thinking Golf is less than lame,
You need to get a life, not just a Game.

James Long Hale

FORGETFULNESS

At my age I've seen it all, done it all and heard it all. I just can't remember it all.

Everyone has a photographic memory. Some just don't have any film.

First you forget names, then you forget faces, then you forget to zip your fly, then you forget to unzip your fly.

Leo Rosenberg

Two elderly guys were discussing great food experiences. One said he went to a fabulous restaurant just last evening. "What was the name of the restaurant?" his friend asked.

"Let me think for a minute. It reminded me of a flower with a green stem and some thorns. Let me call to my wife."

"Rose, what was the name of that restaurant we went to last night?"

– We met at 9.
– We met at 8.
– I was on time.
– No, you were late.
– Ah yes, I remember it well.

Maurice Chevalier
Gigi

My forgetter's getting better,
But my rememberer is broke.
To you that may seem funny,
But to me, that is no joke.

For when I'm 'here' I'm wondering
If I really should be 'there.'
And, when I try to think it through,
I haven't got a prayer!

At times I put something away
Where it is safe, but Gee!
The person it is safest from
Is, generally, me!

When shopping I may see someone,
Say 'Hi' and have a chat,
Then, when the person walks away,
I ask myself, 'who the hell was that?'

FREUD

The great question that has never been answered, and that I have not yet
been able to answer despite my thirty years of research into the feminine
soul, is "What do women want?"

Sigmund Freud

"They want men Sig, but I'm no psychiatrist."

A Freudian Slip Is When You Say One Thing But Mean Your Mother.

Gary Blake
Book Title

An early psychiatrist, Freud,
Had the bluenoses very annoyed,
Saying, "You cannot be rid
Of the troublesome id,
So it might just as well be enjoyed."

FRIEND

…a person we know well enough to borrow from but not well enough to
lend to.

Ambrose Bierce

Old friends are best. They know all about you but can't remember any of it.

You can pick your nose
You can pick your friends
But you cannot pick your friend's nose.

Friend-or-phobia: fear of being asked, "Who goes there?"

I knew the day would come when you would leave me for my best friend.
So here's his leash, water bowl and chew toys.

"Doctor, I'm heading up to rattlesnake country, and I figure I better get a
bit of advice on what to do in case I get bitten by a rattlesnake."
    "Well, if a rattlesnake bites you on the hand, you must immediately
draw the poison out with your mouth and spit out the poison."
    "Yeah, Doc. What if he bites me where I sit down?"
    "That's when you find out who your friends are."

Here's to the friends that I love best,
To those who have always stood the test;
To the friends I love who are tried and true,
Friends that are old, and those that are new.
Life at its best to most is a trial,
'Tis friendship that makes life really worth while.
                                        E.K. Orr

FRUSTRATION
If you could kick the person in the pants responsible for most of your
trouble, you wouldn't sit for a month.
                                        Theodore Roosevelt

There are two appropriate responses to frustration. You can laugh or you
can cry. I prefer laughter because there's less mopping up afterwards.
                                        Kurt Vonnegut

FUN
I never did a day's work in my life — it was all fun.
                                        Thomas A. Edison

It's fundamental in becoming a humor being.

Usually being the right thing in the wrong space and the wrong thing in
the right space is worth it, because something funny always happens.
                                        Andy Warhol
                                        My Philosophy

There ain't much fun in medicine, but there's a heck of a lot of medicine in fun.

Josh Billings
1818-1885

People are funny: they want the front of the bus, the middle of the road and the back of the church.

Silly Impossibilities:
1) You can't count your hair.
2) You can't wash your eyes with soap.
3) You can't breathe when your tongue is out.
    Put your tongue back in your mouth, you silly person.

Things I Know About You:
1) You are reading this.
2) You are human.
3) You can't say the letter "P" without separating your lips.
4) You just attempted to do it.
5) You are laughing at yourself.
6) You laugh at this because you are a fun-loving person.

FUNERALS
...cocktail parties for the geriatric set.

Always go to other people's funerals, otherwise they won't go to yours.

I think we're finally at a point where we've learned to see death with a sense of humor. I have to. When you're my age, it's as if you're a car. First a tire blows, and you get that fixed. Then a headlight goes, and you get that fixed. And then one day, you drive into a shop and the man says, "Sorry, miss, they don't have this make anymore."

Katherine Hepburn

FUNERAL DIRECTOR
...the last guy to let you down.

One funeral director's directives:
Ask about our Lay-Away Plan.
Always keep the fun in funerals.
Why not go out in style?

This eulogy was part of a funeral director's service: "Is there anyone who would like to say a few words on the deceased's behalf?" There was no answer. He asked again. "If anyone would care to say a few words for the dearly beloved, now is the time." After a long pause, a fellow in the back spoke up. "I can tell you this, his brother was worse."

FUNGAL
...a guy's dream; whereas a FUNGI is the answer to that dream. Addendumb: At ease disease, there's fungus among us.

She grew on him like she was a colony of E-coli,
and he was a room-temperature Canadian beef.

Brian Broadus

GASTRIC
...blaming others for your own flatulence.

Astronaut Takes Blame For Gas In Spacecraft.

News headline, 1999

The doctor had to be the bearer of bad news when he told a wife that her husband had died of a massive myocardial infarct. Not more than five minutes later, I heard her reporting to the rest of the family that he had died of a "massive internal fart."

I sat next to the Duchess at tea;
It was just as I had feared it would be;
Her rumblings abdominal
Were truly phenomenal,
And everyone thought it was me.

Woodrow Wilson

GENES
The problem with the gene pool is — there's no lifeguard.

Steven Wright

Scientists have found a gene for shyness. They would have found it years ago, but it was hiding behind a couple of other genes.

Johnathan Katz

GERIATRICS
No one should grow old who isn't ready to appear ridiculous.

John Mortimer

If I'd known I was going to live this long, I'd have taken better care of myself.
Eubie Blake
1883-1983

A man is only as old as he looks. And if he only looks, he's old.

It's the period of life when you buy yourself a see-through night gown, and then remember you don't know anybody who can still see through one.
Betty Davis

As you grow old, you lose interest in sex, your friends drift away, and your children ignore you. There are other advantages, of course, but these are the outstanding ones.
Richard Needham

King David and King Solomon
Led merry, merry lives,
With many, many lady friends
And many, many wives;
But when old age crept over them
With many, many qualms,
King Solomon wrote the Proverbs
And King David wrote the Psalms.

James Ball Naylor

GERMS
...little bugs with influence.

The woman sneezed about 300 times said, "There must be something in the air."
I said, "Yeah, you're germs."
Linda Herskovicly

You have two chances: one of getting the germ and one of not getting the germ. If you get the germ, you have two chances: one of getting the disease, and one of not getting the disease. If you get the disease, you have two chances: one of dying, and one of not dying. And if you die, well, you still have two chances.

GINGIVITIS
...Fred Astaire's dancing partner.

If you think He was great, just remember: Ginger Rogers did everything he did backwards and in high heels.
Addendumb: And we didn't notice Fred's toupee or Ginger's face-lift.

G I SERIES
...soldier's ball game managed by the Upper GI (Top Brass.)

Angry officer: "Not a man in this division will be given liberty this week-end."
Voice in ranks: "Give me liberty or give me death."
Officer: "Who said that?"
Voice: "Patrick Henry."

"While you are away, movie stars are taking your women, Robert Redford is dating your girlfriend, Tom Selleck is kissing your lady, Bart Simpson is making love to your wife."

> *Baghdad Betty, Iraqi Radio*
> (to Gulf War troops)

Fifty-one years ago, Herman James, a North Carolina mountain man, was drafted by the army. On his first day in basic training, the army issued him a comb. That afternoon the Army barber sheared off all his hair. On his second day, the army issued Herman a toothbrush. That afternoon the army dentist yanked seven of his teeth. On the third day, the Army issued him a jock strap. The army has been looking for Herman for 51 years.

GLUTEUS MAXIMUS
...best if kept to a minimus.

I used to have a big barrel chest, but that's all behind me now.
> Bob Hope

Childhood obesity slogan: Leave No Child With A Big Behind.
> Bill Novelli

GLUTTON
Mea gulpa, mea gulpa, mea maxima gulpa.

The influence of affluence
Makes this a land where fester all
The gluttonous diseases that
Are festered by cholesterol.
These coronary carriers

Evade the pampered foreigner;
Prosperity, it seems to me,
Is just around the corner.

E.Y."Yip" Harburg

(Or just around the coroner)

GOLD THERAPY (Auranofin)
...a flash in the pan.

This condition has caused an outbreak of gold pandemonium at some hospitals.

GOSSIP
...a fool with a keen sense of rumor.

It's nothing more than mouth-to-mouth recitation.

A gossip is one who talks to you about other people.
A bore is one who talks to you about himself.
A brilliant conversationalist is one who talks to you about yourself.

Dr. William King

Show me someone who never gossips,
and I'll show you someone who isn't interested in people.

Barbara Walters

Uttermost: the worst gossiper.

Gossip is the most deadly microbe,
It has neither legs nor wings,
It is composed mostly of tales
And most of them have stings.

E. E. Opdyke

GRAN MAL SEIZURES
...condition caused by over-zealous shoppers.

Once you've seen one shopping center, you've seen a mall.

Buy-ology: Some swear that "Shop till you drop" is a real stress-buster.

Best advice: When shopportunity knocks, don't answer it.

GYNECOLOGIST
...a doctor who puts in a hard day at the orifice and can be a spreader of old wives tales.

A male gynecologist is like an auto mechanic who has never owned a car.
                                                    Carrie Snow

Malady: female disorder.

I've always wanted to date a gynecologist. I want to know I'm special.
                                                    Jane Christie Coupling

HAIR
...is often hair today and gone tomorrow.

What he hath scanted men in hair, he hath given them in wit.
                                                    William Shakespeare
                                                    Comedy of Errors

Hippocrates noted that eunuchs never lost their hair. This remains one of the few potential cures for hair loss that never caught on.

Alopecia: a low Hawaiian hair chant.
                                                    N.H.

Once I was standing on a hill, my hair blowing in the breeze, but I was too embarrassed to run after it.

Hair is a constant problem with men and women.
With women it's the tint and with men it's the t'aint.
                                                    Herm Albright

HALITOSIS
...a breath that takes yours away.

Lockjaw: a halitosis remedy.

Mahatma Gandhi walked barefoot everywhere, to the point where the soles of his feet became quite thick and hard. Being a very spiritual person, he ate very little and often fasted. As a result, he was quite thin and frail. Furthermore, due to his diet, he ended up with very bad breath. Therefore, he came to be known as a super-callused-fragile-mystic-plagued-with-halitosis.

HAPPINESS

When one door of happiness closes, another opens; but often we look so long at the closed door that we do not see the other one which has been opened to us.

> Helen Keller
> 1880-1968

It's having a scratch for every itch.

> Ogden Nash

The road to happiness is always under construction.

It's watching TV at your girlfriend's house during a power failure.
> Bob Hope

A good cigar, a good meal, and a good woman — or a bad woman. It depends on how much happiness you can handle.
> George Burns

For every minute you are angry, you lose 60 seconds of happiness.
> Ralph Waldo Emerson

Addendum: My psychologist told me to pick just one person in the world to make happy. I picked me.

Secrets to a long happy marriage: An old woman sipping a glass of wine on the patio with her husband, and she says, "I love you so much, I don't know how I could ever live without you." Her husband asks, "Is that you or the wine talking?" She replies, "It's me… and I'm talking to the wine!"

HEALTH

Good health and good sense are two great blessings.
> *Latin Proverb*

It's no longer a question of staying healthy.
It a question of finding a sickness you like.
> Jackie Mason

Sooner or later everything we've heard about staying healthy turns out to be wrong. They'll probably decide chicken soup is bad for you.
> Andy Rooney

Health nuts are going to feel stupid someday, lying in a hospital bed dying of nothing.
> Redd Foxx

I drink to your health when I'm with you,
I drink to your health when I'm alone,
I drink to your health so often
I'm beginning to worry about my own.

HEALTH ADVICE

Don't sit on your fatty acids.

Irvine Page, M.D.

The only way to keep your health is to eat what you don't want,
drink what you don't like and do what you'd rather not.

Mark Twain

Last week I went to my doctor for my annual physical. Things are looking
up for me. My weight is up, my blood pressure is up, my PSA is up and
my cholesterol is up.

Doctor to patient:
"Sure, laughter is the best medicine — but Cialis is a very close second."

If you receive an e-mail from the Department of Health telling you not to
eat pork because of swine flu, ignore it. It's just Spam.

HEALTH FOOD

Health food makes me sick.

Calvin Trillin

Half of what you eat keeps you alive; the other half kills you.

Henny Youngman

Have you ever seen the customers in health-food stores?
They are pale, skinny people who look half dead.
In a steak house, you see robust, ruddy people.
They're dying, of course, but they look terrific.

Bill Cosby

HEALTH PREVENTION

Mary had a little cold, but wouldn't stay at home,
And everywhere that Mary went, the cold was sure to roam.
It wandered into Molly's eyes and filled them full of tears.
It jumped from there to Bobby's nose and thence to Jimmie's ears.
It painted Anna's throat bright red, and swelled poor Jennie's head.

Dora had a fever, and cough put Jack to bed.
The moral of this little tale is very quickly said.
Mary could have saved great pain with just one day in bed.

HEART
A merry heart doeth good like a medicine.
Proverbs 17:22

She was wearing a low-cut gown, but you could tell her heart wasn't in it.

The way to a man's heart may be through his stomach, but the way to a
woman's heart is through the door of a good restaurant.
Elliot Joseph
McCalls

Doctor to garage mechanic in his own language:
"You have a slow leak in your lower chamber requiring a valve job."

Triple Bypass: when a guy hits a three-bagger and forgets to step on second
base.
Johnny Hart
B.C.

"Would you please turn on the TV.
I'd like to see if I am still alive and how I'm doing."
Murray Haydon
Artificial heart recipient

HEMORRHOIDS
Seven out of ten people suffer from hemorrhoids.
Do the other three enjoy them?

Analyst: a hemorrhoid specialist who believes that half of all analysis is anal.

A shrink a day keeps the doctor away.

They won't kill you. You just wish they would.
Addendumb: "Mr. Pharmist, do ya have any supprisatories for hammerrids?"

Hemorrhoids are a pain in the – – –,
To scratch them in public demonstrates no class.
Showing them to doctors is very embarrassing.
I'd rather treat them with Plaster of Paris-ing.

And nothing I find, in public offends
As seeing a panty bulge — Depends.
Hemorrhoids (I believe to be on the level)
Weren't made by God, but by the devil.

Joel Berman M.D.

HISTORY
Humor is like history. It repeats itself.

History is more or less bunk.

Henry Ford

Grant stood by me when I was crazy, and I stood by him when he was
drunk, and now we stand by each other.

General William T. Sherman

According to one researcher, Alexander The Great whipped up a crude
time-piece for his soldiers consisting of a chemically treated cloth worn on
the left forearm. Under the heat of the sun, the cloth changed colors every
hour, providing the Macedonian warriors with the world's first wrist watch.
Among historians the device is known as "Alexander's Rag Time Band."

Even Napoleon had his Watergate.

Yogi Berra

One of the world's oldest recorded jokes is a 1600 BC gag about a pharaoh
named King Snofru — "How do you entertain a bored pharaoh? You sail a
boatload of young women dressed only in fishing nets down the Nile and
urge the pharaoh to go catch a fish."

HMO
…Help Me Out

Early to bed and early to arise, just might keep your health premium alive.

I finally have a dental plan. I chew on the other side.

Janine Ditullio

Doctor to patient: Of course, a full-body scan can be done more cheaply if
you go through airport security.
Addendumb: And the best breast exams could be conducted at Hooters.

Patient: My job is giving me migraines, high blood pressure, chest pains, and ulcers.
Doctor: Why don't you quit?
Patient: Are you kidding. I have a fabulous health plan.

The AMA on national health insurance:
Allergists voted to scratch it.
Dermatologists advised not to make any rash moves.
Gastroenterologists had sort of a gut feeling about it.
Neurologists thought the Administration had a lot of nerve.
Obstetricians felt they were all laboring under a misconception.
Ophthalmologists considered the idea shortsighted.
Pathologists yelled, "Over my dead body!"
Pediatricians said, "Oh, grow up."
Psychiatrists thought the whole idea was madness.
Radiologists could see right through it.
Surgeons decided to wash their hands of the whole thing.
Internists thought it was a bitter pill to swallow.
Plastic surgeons said, "This puts a whole new face on the matter."
Podiatrists thought it was a step forward.
Urologists were pissed off at the whole idea.
Anesthesiologists thought the whole idea was a gas.
Cardiologists didn't have the heart to say no.

HOMEOPATHY
...dilutions of grandeur.

The homeopathic system, sir,
Just suits me to a tittle.
It proves of physic anyhow,
You cannot take too little.
If it be good in any case
To take a dose so small,
It surely must be better still
To take no dose at all.

HOMO SAPIENS
...the only animal with brains to find a cure for the diseases caused by his own folly.

I wished I loved the human race;
I wished I loved its silly face;
I wished I loved the way it walks;
I wished I loved the way it talks;
And when I'm introduced to one,
I wish I thought *what jolly fun.*

Sir Walter Raleigh

HOSPITAL
...a place where a private room has nothing to do with privacy.

It's like a convent, the hospital. You leave the world behind and take vows of poverty, chastity, and obedience.

Carolyn Wheat

Hospital bed: a parked taxi with the meter running.

Groucho Marx

Hospital on a budget: Instead of a sponge bath, they send in a Saint Bernard to lick you all over. The dog is great company and has an extra elixir under his neck.

N.H.

HOSPITAL CHARTS:
Patient is to remain plastered for the next six to eight weeks.

The patient is a smoker, so will be admitted to a smoking bed.

While in the ER, she was examined, X-rated and sent home.

Ever since Mrs. Wilson had her gallbladder removed,
she can't tolerate greasy males. I mean meals.

She has had no rigors or shaking chills,
but her husband states that she was really hot in bed last night.

HOSPITAL GOWN
...the end of hospitality.

The first thing you learn from a hospital stay is that you're not fully covered by the insurance or your gown.

Have patience, will travel: Patient's gowns are open in back because they are easily accessible and are I-C-U gowns.

HOSPITALIZATION PREPARATION
I was taken to the hospital for observation.
I stayed several days, didn't observe anything, and left.
George Carlin

Lay on the front lawn dressed in paper napkins with straws stuck up your nose and ask people to poke you as they go by.
Kathryn Hammer
How Are We Feeling Today?

HUG
... releases oxytocin, the "love hormone" that quells anxiety.

Some think it is just energy gone to waist.

Being hugged by Diana Riggs is worth three sessions of chemotherapy.
Robert Runcie

It's a round-about way of expressing affection.
Addendumb: or a sound about way — "If someone said you have a nice body, would you hold that against them?"

HUMOR
...emotional chaos remembered in tranquility.
James Thurber

God is a great humorist, but He has a slow audience.
Garrison Keillor

It's important to know the difference between humor and odor.
Humor is when you shift your wit — odor is the other way around.
Patty Wooten, R.N.
Nancy Nurse

If you think you're a wit, make sure you're not half right.
Addendumb: But if you laugh your head off, it's a great way to go.

Alphabetically speaking — I'm OK.
A is for apple, and B is for boat, that used to be right, but now it won't float.
Age before beauty is what we once said, but let's be a bit more realistic instead.
Now A's for arthritis;
B's the bad back,
C is for chest pains, perhaps cardiac.
D is for dental decay and decline;
E is for eyesight, can't read that top line.
F is for fissures and fluid retention,
G is for gas, which I'd rather not mention.
H is high blood pressure. I'd rather it low;
I for incisions with scars you can show.
J is for joints, out of socket, won't mend.
K is for knees that crack when they bend.
L for libido, what happened to sex?
M is for memory. I forget what comes next.
N is neuralgia, in nerves way down low.
O is for osteo, the bones that won't grow!
P for prescriptions, I have quite a few, Just give me a pill and I'll be good as new.
Q is for queasy, is it fatal or flu?
R for reflux, one meal turns to two.
S for sleepless nights, counting my fears.
T for tinnitus, there's bells in my ears.
U is for urinary, big troubles with flow,
V is for vertigo, that's "dizzy" you know.
W is for worry, now what's going around.
X is for X-ray, and what might be found.
Y is another year I'm left here behind.
Z is for zest that I still have — in my mind.

I've survived all the symptoms, my body's deployed, and I've kept twenty-six doctors fully employed! May your troubles be less, your blessings more, and nothing but happiness come through your door.

Humor is not a condiment;
It's a main course.
It's not a trinket;
It's a gem.
It doesn't need justification;
It's essential.

HYPOCHONDRIAC
...one who wants to have his ache and treat it too,
and believes life is a bed of neuroses.

He always feels bad when he feels good for fear he'll feel worse when he feels better.

Organ recital: a hypochondriac's medical history.

Hypochondria cure: The best cure is to forget about your body and get interested in someone else's.

Goodman Ace

First, I got angina pectoris and then arteriosclerosis. Just as I recovering from these, I got tuberculosis and double pneumonia. Then they gave me hypodermics. Appendicitis was followed by tonsillectomy. These gave way to aphasia and hypertrophic cirrhosis. I completely lost my memory for a while. I know I had diabetes and acute indigestion, besides gastritis, rheumatism and neuritis.

I don't know how I managed to survive. It was the hardest spelling test I'd ever had.

Stomach trouble, headache pain,
Is he truly a believer
In his hurt, or does he feign?
Can some secret, keen dislike be
Something he considers hid?
Does he have a shaky psyche?
Does his ego mock his id?
In short, is he actually stricken,
Or — just chicken?

H. Louis Hermance

INCOMPATIBILITY
…when a drug loses its income and patent ability.

N.H.

Of people: I believe a little incompatibility is the spice of life, particularly if he has income and she is pattable.

Ogden Nash

Do you think they're incompatible?
He's on Ritalin and she's on Prozac.
They say "opposites attract."

He has a future and I have a past, so we should be all right.

Jennie Churchill

INDIGESTION
...is charged by God with enforcing morality on the stomach.

Victor Hugo

Dyspepsia: a stomach ache brought on by drinking one Pepsi too many.

He had such tenacity after he won "The Pants On Fire" award in the chili run-off.

...a disease which the patient and his friends frequently mistake for the deep religious conviction and concern for the salvation of all mankind. As the simple Red Man of the western wild put it, with it must be confessed a certain force: "Plenty well, no pray; big belly ache, heap God."

Ambrose Bierce

INDULGENT
...a man who has worked his way down from "bottoms up."

'Twas an evening in November
And I very well remember
I was walking down the street in drunken pride.
But my knees were all aflutter,
So I landed in the gutter,
And a pig came up and lay down by my side.
Yes, I lay there in the gutter
Thinking thoughts I could not utter,
When a girl passing by did softly say,
"You can tell a man that boozes
By the company he chooses."
At that the pig got up and walked away.

INFATUATE
... is equal to in-fat-u-die.

Has it ever struck you that there's a thin person inside of every fat one, just as they say there's a statue inside every block of stone?

George Orwell

If you want to stay healthy, give up those intimate little dinners for two unless you have someone to share them with.

Infatuation: when men lean toward big women, but not enough to alter their stance.

Now I lay me down to sleep,
I pray the Lord my shape to keep.
Please no wrinkles, please no bags
And please lift my butt before it sags.
Please no age spots, please no gray,
And as for my belly, please take it away.
Please keep me healthy, please keep me young,
And thank you Dear Lord for all you've done.

INNUENDO
...an Italian suppository.

From angry patient: For all the good they did me, I could have shoved them up my "you know what."

INSANITY
...doing the same thing over and over and expecting different results.
                                                    Benjamin Franklin

We go by majority vote. If the majority are insane, the sane must go to the hospital.
                                                    Horace Mann
                                                    1796-1859

Insanity runs in my family. It practically gallops.
                                                    Cary Grant
                                                    Arsenic and Old Lace

When his patron complained of a pain,
The pharmacist said with disdain:
"To take medication
For hallucination
Would be absolutely insane."

INSOMNIA
...a person who can't sleep because he worries about it and worries about it because he can't sleep.
                                                    Franklin P. Adams
Addendumb: The cure? Lie on the edge of the bed until you drop off.

Perched in my shorts on the edge of my bed,
With a shoe in my hand and my teeth in a cup,
I'm looking for clues, so I don't have to ask:
Am I going to bed now or just getting up?

Jane Thomas Nolan

INTERCOURSE
...a friendly conversation to some and a gland finale to others.

Before sleeping together today, people should boil themselves.

Richard Lewis

A doctor asked an old gentleman during his interview, "Sir, do you have intercourse?"

The patient looked bewildered and thought for a moment. "You know, I don't know. I'll have to ask my wife." He then stood up, went to the waiting room and located his wife. "Honey, do we have intercourse?" The wife responded with indignation, "Herman, I've told you and told you, we have Blue Cross Blue Shield."

INTERNS
...practicing until they get it right.

They scare me. They're too young. How can you have confidence in a doctor who has his rubber gloves pinned to his sleeves.

Joan Rivers

JOCULAR
...sports minded.

Water polo: I quit this after the horse drowned.

Water skiing: a rich man's enema. I tried it once but couldn't get the boat up the hill.

The mold out of which good skiers are cast is usually plaster of paris.

Art Buchwald

Basketball is the second most exciting sport, and the other one shouldn't have spectators.

Dick Vertleib

I should warn you that under these clothes I'm wearing boxer shorts
and I know how to use them.

Obert Orben

Tug McGraw was asked if he pitched better on Astroturf or grass.
His response was "I don't know. I've never smoked Astroturf."

I doubt that I should ever view
Another football game with you.
You holler nonstop in my ear
For every tackle makes you cheer,
Or bellow in a wounded way,
Depending on who makes the play.
I do not understand the charm
Of watching athletes doing harm.
Football's played for fools like you,
But I have better things to do.

JOCKSTRAP
...a ballpark.

Some men aren't sports minded, but they are athletic supporters.

When Sir John Gielgud told the Shakespearean actors that all the men
must wear jockstraps under their leotards, a player asked, "Please, Sir John,
does that apply to those of us who only have small parts?"

KIDNEY
...a youngsters leg joint.

Patient: Doctor, I can't seem to hold my water lately.
        What do you suggest that I do?
Doctor: Well, the very first thing,
        please step off my new carpeting without delay.

Kidney Dialysis: It's like being connected to a washing machine.

Art Buchwald

Kidney Stones: personal pet rocks.

There was a fellow named Sydney,
Who drank till he ruined his kidney.
It shriveled and shrank
As he sat there and drank,
But he'd had a good time at it, didn'he?

KIDS
Nothing you do for children is wasted.

Garrison Keillor

Two boys were bragging about their parents:
"My Dad is a doctor. I can be sick for nothing."
"Well, my Dad is a minister. I can be good for nothing."

A mother had been lecturing her small son that we are in this world to
help others.
    He considered this, then asked somberly, "What are others here for?"

Asking a young boy what was the best way to preserve milk, he said,
"Keep it in the cow."

Child letter to the Almighty: Dear God, Instead of letting people die and
having to make new ones, Why don't you just keep the ones you have now.

Jamie

Two kindergarten kids were discussing religion.
"If Christ is Jesus last name, what is God's last name?"
"I got it. It's God Dammit!"

A little boy said to his teacher, "I ain't got no pencil!"
    She corrected him at once: "It's I don't have a pencil. You don't have a
pencil. We don't have any pencils. Is that clear?"
    "No!" said the boy. "What happened to all those pencils?"

KISS
...lip service.

It's a contraction of the mouth due to an enlargement of the heart.

If you are ever in doubt as to whether or not you should kiss a pretty girl,
always give her the benefit of the doubt.

Thomas Carlyle

Stealing a kiss may be petty larceny, but usually it's grand.

People who throw kisses are hopelessly lazy.
Bob Hope

I'd love to kiss you, but I just washed my hair.
Bette Davis
Cabin in the Cotton

I do love the rain so. It reminds me of my first kiss.
Ah, your first kiss was in the rain?
No, it was in the shower.
Blanche and Dorothy
The Golden Girls
Pssst: The girls are off their rocker. It was at a garden baby shower.

The doctor must have given me a faulty pacemaker.
When my husband kisses me the garage door goes up.
Minnie Pearl

Liposuction: a kissing disease.

Oh, innocent victim of Cupid,
Remember this terse little verse:
To let a fool kiss you is stupid,
To let a kiss fool you is worse.

E.Y. "Yip" Harburg

LANGUAGE
Laughter is the universal language.

Two highway workers are at a construction site when a car with diplomatic plates pulls up. "Parles-vous francais?" the driver asks. The two just stare. "Hablam ustedes espanol?" the driver tries. They stare some more. "Sprechen Se Deutsch?" They continue to stare. "Parle Italiano?" Nothing. Finally the man drives off in disgust.

One worker turns to the other and says, "Maybe we should learn a foreign language." "What for?" the other replies. "That guy knew four of them, and a lot of good it did him."
Maxime Cosma

"Did I mention I was flatulent in many languages?"
From a 6th grader

"Gesundheit!"—The answer to the common cold.

The Norwegian language has been described as German spoken underwater.

Gaffes Around the World:
Mexican Brochure — Come to Juan's Jewelry Shop.
    We won't screw you too much.
Cairo Tourist Office Ad for a donkey ride —
    Would you like to ride on your own ass?
Tel Aviv Hotel — For room breakfast, waitress will arrive.
    This will bring your food up.
In Istanbul shop window — Sorry, We Are Open.
At Thailand Laundromat — For Best Results, Drop Pants Here.
Taiwan sign — Mens Underware. They're Comfartable.
Moscow hotel lobby — If this is your first visit to the USSR,
    you are welcome to it.
On Chinese Train — Please do not throw yourself out the window.

Hey, Shakespeare!
If all the world's a stage,
What are we To Be or do
Who oft confuse the two,
And sadly for those few
Meandering through your Much Ado?

                                        N.H.

LAUGHTER
With the fearful strain that is on me night and day,
if I did not laugh I should die.

                                        Abraham Lincoln

It's America's most important export.

                                        Walt Disney

Laughter is an interior convulsion producing a distortion of the features
and accompanied by inarticulate noises. It is infectious and, though
intermittent, incurable.

                                        Ambrose Bierce

Laffing iz the sensation of pheeling good all over,
and show'n it principally in one spot.

                                        Josh Billings
                                        1818-1895

It's like a pesticide. Use it on everyone that bugs you.

N.H.

Laugh and the whole world laughs with you. Cry and you cry alone.
Laugh alone and they lock you up.

Steve Kissell

I am thankful for laughter, except when milk comes out of my nose.

Woody Allen

He/she who laughs last, laughs alone.
Or doesn't get it.

The limerick packs laughs anatomical
Into space that is quite economical.
But the good ones I've seen
So seldom are clean
And the clean ones so seldom are comical.

LAUGHING STOCK
These are more than contented cows.
They are cattle with a great sense of humor.

Never approach a bull from the front, a horse from the rear, or a fool from
any direction.

Danny Saradon

Udder nonsense: "The cow jumped over the moon."

A farmer was asked how much milk his cows gave. He answered,
"My cows don't give no milk — I gotta take it from them."

Ah, yes, I wrote the Purple Cow.
I'm sorry now, I wrote it!
But I can tell you anyhow,
I'll kill you if you quote it.

Gelett Burgess

LAXITY
...poor bowel habits.

The general practitioner's association with the bowels begins with the digestion of large amounts of information at medical school. Quite often the intellectual nutrition is in a high fiber form; much of it is unabsorbed and goes straight through.

Cliff Hawkins
Alimentary, My Dear

You've got to wonder if anyone proof reads those ads on TV. Last night I saw this laxative ad where the main selling point was that the stuff works while you sleep. That doesn't sound too wonderful to me.

Ron Dentinger

"I've been constipated for weeks," said Mrs. Shaw.
"What are you doing for it?" her doctor asked.
"Well, I'm sitting on the toilet an hour a day."
"No, I mean what do you take?"
"Oh," Mrs. Shaw said, "I take my knitting."

LAZINESS
...hardening of the oughteries.

Who says nothing is impossible? I've been doing nothing all day.
Addendumb: How do you know when you're done doing nothing?

It is better to have loafed and lost than never to have loafed at all.

James Thurber
Fables For Our Time

Dust if you must, but wouldn't it be better,
To paint a picture or write a letter,
Bake a cake or plant a seed,
Ponder the difference between want and need?

Dust if you must, but there's not much time,
With rivers to swim and mountains to climb,
Music to hear and books to read,
Friends to cherish and life to lead.

Dust if you must, but the world's out there,
With the sun in your eyes, and the wind in your hair,
A flutter of snow, a shower of rain.
This day will not come 'round again.

Dust if you must, but bear in mind,
Old age will come and it's not always kind.
And when you go and go you must,
You, yourself, will make more dust.

LIFE
The unexamined life is not worth living.

> Socrates
> *Plato's Apology*
> *c.399 B.C.*

Life is what happens to you while you are making other plans.

> Thomas la Mance

The world is a grindstone and life is your nose.

> Fred Allen

I hope life is not some big joke, because I don't get it.

If life deals you lemons, make lemonade.
If it deals you tomatoes, make Bloody Marys.

The stages of life:
To grow up.
To fill out.
To slim down.
To hold it in.
To heck with it.

A slice of life:
If life is a waste of time, and time is a waste of life, then let's all get wasted together and have the time of our lives.

> *Armand's Pizza*
> *Washington, DC*

Life is not a bowl of cherries. It is a bowl of fizzing Alka Selzers.
Addendumb: And we're just innocent bubbles.

What is Success in Life?
At age 4…success is…not peeing in your pants.
At age 12...success is…having friends.
At age 16...success is…having a driver's license.
At age 20...success is…having sex.
At age 35...success is…having money.

At age 50...success is...having money.
At age 60...success is...having sex.
At age 70...success is...having a driver's license.
At age 80...success is...not peeing in your pants.

Phil Proctor

LIFESTYLE
I just use my muscles as a conversation piece,
like someone walking a cheetah down 42nd Street.

Arnold Schwarzenegger

If you can start the day without caffeine or pep pills,
If you can be cheerful, ignoring aches and pains,
If you can resist complaining and boring people with your troubles,
If you can eat the same food every day and be grateful for it,
If you can understand when loved ones are too busy to give you time,
If you can forgive those who take things out on you,
If you can take criticism and blame without resentment,
If you can face the world without lies and deceit,
If you can conquer tension without medical help,
If you can relax without liquor,
If you can sleep without the aid of drugs,
If you can do all of these things,
Then you are probably the family dog.

LIQUIDATE
...cocktails for two.

Bourbon: a corny liquid, containing sugar and alcohol. The corn gives you courage, the sugar gives you energy, and the alcohol gives you ideas on what to do with all that courage and energy.

I was on a date with this really hot model. Well, it wasn't really a date-date. We just ate dinner and saw a movie. Then the plane landed.

Dave Attell

PS: At the terminal she had something else that would knock your eyes out — a husband.

LIVER
Is life worth living? It depends on the liver.

William James

Liver Pills:
An old man I know, name of Frick,
Took liver pills to avoid being sick.
He died quite old,
But his liver I'm told,
Had to be beaten to death with a stick.

Ode to Carter Little

LOBOTOMY
Better a free bottle in front of me than a prefrontal lobotomy.
Dorothy Parker

Wouldn't that be a great name for a prostate operation — a low-botomy?
Robert Orben

I drink when I'm happy and when I'm sad. Sometimes, I drink when I'm alone. When I have company, I consider it obligatory. I trifle with it when I'm not hungry and drink it when I am. Otherwise, I never touch it — unless I'm thirsty.

Lily Bollinger

LONGEVITY
He who laughs, lasts.

Mary Pettibone Poole

You're a positive friend for life extension.
You eat greens in every dimension.
You know as well as any parrot
The quirks of calorie and carrot.
They've taken out without a quiver,
Your tonsils, teeth, ambition, liver,
Appendix, income — every center
Designed to let bacilli enter.
You never miss the daily dozen
That killed your uncle, brother, cousin.
You breathe only the fresh breezes
And what do you get? The same diseases.

Samuel Hoffenstein
1890-1947

LOVE
…a grave mental disease.

Plato

One is very crazy when in love.
>
> Sigmund Freud

"Sig, I'm a — Freud you lost me on that one."

Love cures people — both the ones who give it and the ones who receive it.
>
> Carl Menninger M.D.

When the moon hits your eye like a big pizza pie, *That's Amore.*
>
> Dean Martin
> *1953 hit song*

No matter how lovesick a woman is, she shouldn't take the first pill who comes along.
>
> Dr. Joyce Brothers

It is better to have loved and lost than to spend the rest of your life with a psycho.
>
> Dr. Phil

Addendumb: It is also better to have loved a short person than to never have loved a tall.

Life is just one fool thing after another,
while love is just two fool things after each other.
>
> Frank Moore Colby

Do you know what it means to come home at night to a woman who'll give you a little love, a little affection, a little tenderness?
It means you're in the wrong house, that's what it means.
>
> Henny Youngman

Your little hands,
Your little feet,
Your little mouth —
Oh God, how sweet!
Your little nose,
Your little ears,
Your eyes that shed
Such little tears!
Your little voice,
So soft and kind;
Your little soul,
Your little mind!

>
> Samuel Hoffenstein
> *Love-Songs*

"Sam! To belittle is to be little."

MAGIC BULLET
...a drug that hits the target but spares the patient.
Addendumb: Not to be confused with a super suppository.

Miracle drug: Any medicine you can get the kids to take without screaming.

Wonder drug: You never know what's going to happen, so don't wander too far.

MA HUANG (Ephedra sineca)
...the mother of all drugs. Used in China for 5000 years.
No one knows who the father is.

A single untried popular remedy throws the scientific doctor into hysterics.
Chinese Proverb

Asking for Ma Huang when I was in China in 2006, the clerk knew
where to find it. Our tour guide Yee Wong liked the way Americans used
the good news-bad news concept in telling a story, so he tried it on us:
"I know you Americans are more than ready for a good swim. At the
next stop there is a pool." Cheers went up. "That's the good news.
The bad news is, there's no water in the pool."

MAMMOGRAM
...a test to keep you abreast.

Every time I hear it, I think I'm supposed to put my breast in an envelope
and send it to someone.

Jan King

MASTECTOMY:
It hasn't changed my lifestyle
And I haven't lost my touch.
The only thing I find is,
I don't skinny-dip as much

Janet Henry

MARIJUANA (Cannabis sativa)
...a trance plant.

Do you believe in the medical use of marijuana? A college newspaper
recently suggested that the marijuana question could easily be settled by
a joint session of Congress.

Who fits in anymore? I was invited to a pot party and I brought Tupperware.

Joan Rivers

When asked what he would like to see on his tomb: "Keep off the grass."

Peter Ustinov

News item: The Straight Dope/Don't Expect Your Physician to Say "Smoke Two Joints, and Call Me in the Morning."

Arizona Republic, 1999

Glass Blower's Demise
Once there was a man of class
Who loved to blow glass and grass,
Inhaling 'till he became insane,
His legacy remains a stomach pane.

N.H.

MARRIAGE
…is a union that defies management.

It's like vitamins: We supplement each other's minimum daily requirements.

Kathy Mohnke

A very brief history of marriage:
Niagra 1963
Viagra 1999

Judith Viorst

I was married by a judge. I should have asked for a jury.

Groucho Marx

If it's true that girls are inclined to marry men like their fathers, it's understandable why so many mothers cry so much at weddings.

A wife asked her husband. "What do you like most in me, my pretty face or my sexy body?"
    He looked at her from head to toe and replied, "I like your sense of humor."

I never married because there was no need. I have three pets at home which answer the same purpose as a husband. I have a dog that growls every morning, a parrot that swears all afternoon, and a cat that comes home late at night.

Marie Corelli

Wife: In most marriage ceremonies, they don't use the word "obey" now.
Husband: Too bad, isn't it? It used to add a little humor to the occasion.

She was married to a banker, an actor, a minister and an undertaker.
It was one for the money, two for the show, three to get ready and four to go.

To keep your marriage brimming
With love in the loving cup,
Whenever you're wrong, admit it;
Whenever you're right, shut up.

                                        Ogden Nash

MASSAGE
...really old.

Nothing beats a good rub.

If you are irritated by every rub, how will your mirror be polished?
                                        Rumi (1207-1273)
                                        Persian poet and philosopher

MASTURBATION
...the sin of emission.

I don't even masturbate anymore. I'm so afraid I'll give myself something.
I just want to be friends with myself.
                                        Richard Lewis

A study in Italy showed that people who eat a lot of pizza are less likely to
get colon cancer. And another study says masturbation reduces risk of
prostate cancer. It's what I've always said: diet and exercise.
                                        Jay Leno

MEDICAL BOOKS
I went to a bookstore today. I asked the woman behind the counter where
the self-help section is.
    She said, "If I told you, that would defeat the whole purpose."

A fellow had been doctoring himself out of a medical book for many years
finally succumbed. He died of a misprint.

MEDICAL ECONOMICS

Always laugh when you can. It is cheap medicine.

Lord Byron
English Poet

A hospital should also have a recovery room adjoining the cashier's office.

Francis O'Walsh

Mother: Don't you think, doctor, you've rather overcharged for attending Jimmy when he had the measles?
Doctor: You must remember, Mrs. Brown, that includes three visits.
Mother: Yes, but you forgot. He infected the whole school.

At drug counter: The bad news sir, is that this prescription is 120 dollars.
Patient: What's the good news?
"No refills."

Doc said he'd have me on my feet
The last time I was ill.
And so he did. I sold my car
So I could pay his bill.

MEDICAL GRAFFITI CHRONOLOGY

1940s — You spend one night with Venus and then a lifetime with Mercury.
1950s — Penicillin took the sin out of syphilis.
1960s — Give me Librium or give me Meth.
1970s — Discretion is the better part of Valium.
1980s — Real Coke is the thing.
1990s — Give me Prozac or give me probate.
2000s — Viagra — Be all you can be.
2010s — Oxymortoxy

MEDICAL HISTORY

2000 BC: Here, eat this root.
1000 BC: That root is heathen. Say this prayer.
1850 AD: That prayer is superstition. Here, drink this potion.
1940 AD: That potion is snake oil. Here, swallow this pill.
1985 AD: That pill is ineffective. Here, take this antibiotic.
2000 AD: That antibiotic doesn't work anymore. Here, eat this root.

The Ecologist

Why do I run? 'Tain't no mystery,
Wanna have a good medical history.
Doctor told me runnin' is great,
Helps them blood cells circulate.
Great for the lungs, great for the ticker,
Can't nothin' getcha in better shape quicker.
Feels so healthy, feels so sweet,
Pumpin' and flappin' my feet.
Moldin' my muscles, firmin' my form,
Pantin'like a pack mule, sweatin'up a storm.
Keeps me youthful, keeps me loose,
Tightens my tummy and shrinks my caboose.
Beats bein' sluggish, beats bein' lazy,
Why do I run? Maybe I'm crazy!

Scott Ross

MEDICAL RESEARCHERS
They have discovered a new disease that has no symptoms. It is impossible to detect, and there is no known cure. Fortunately, no cases have been reported so far.

George Carlin

Hypothesis: A research paper on vaccination.

A new drug is coming out that is the most potent of its kind so far.
The trouble is you can't take it, unless you're in perfect health.

MEDICAL SPECIALIZATION
The practice of medicine today is so specialized that each doctor is a healer of one disease and no more.

Herodotus
c.430 B.C.

It has reached such a state today that patients have to learn to diagnose themselves before they know which specialist to call.

Two Minutes With You

Specialists keep shorter hours.
Door sign: Dr. Doolittle — 9 to 1.
After reading this, the man said, "With odds like that, I'll take care of myself."

Oncologist: a doctor who never keeps you waiting.

An internist is someone who knows everything and does nothing.
A surgeon is someone who does everything and knows nothing.
A pathologist is someone who knows everything and does everything too late.

MEDICINE CHEST
It doesn't take an oxymoron to know. It is well stacked or well stocked.

How about those medicine bottle caps suddenly turning into Rubik's Cubes?

From the Nature's Medicine Chest catalogue you can order:
Green Magma, Ghee, Bio Salt, Carbon Steel, Rhino Chewie Bits, Garlic
Ear Drops, Goodbye Bugs Sun Block, Lady "V" Pleasure Pills, Dream
Cream, Unscented Aural, Glow Oil, Wild Yam Balancing Ointment,
Masad Dead Sea Foot Scrub, Royal Jelly Boosters, Kitchen Sprouters,
Vegetable Crisper Bags and Roto Juicers, and Cat's Claw Intestinal
Cleanser. Truly homeopathic.

> Phil Proctor
> *Funny Times*

I felt that the assortment of tablets that I had been given may have been
mis-prescribed, since they seem to interfere with the pleasant effects of
alcohol. In the interests of my health, therefore, I stopped taking them.

> Barry Humphries

Rogers and Hammerstein (Revisited)
My Favorite Things:
Zyrtec and Zantac and hydroxine,
These are a few of my favorite things.
Eye drops and nose drops to get through the day,
Thank God for insurance or I couldn't pay!
When the nose drips…
When the eyes clot,
When your sneeze your nose away,
Remember to take your meds every day,
And then you won't feeeeel so bad.

> Mark Clark R.N.

MEDITATION
…an affordable medicine.

The nice thing about meditation is that it makes doing nothing quite
respectable.

> Paul Dean

My Dad believed in meditation. He used to tell me, "Sit down and shut up!"

MEN
MENtal breakdown, MENopause, MENstrual cramps, MENtal fatigue
— lots of women's problems begin with MEN.

Dorothy Stauffer, R.N.

If women dressed for men, the stores wouldn't sell much —
just an occasional sun visor.

Groucho Marx

Male menopause: the time when a man starts to turn off the lights for
economic rather than romantic reasons.

Jon Merino

Men are from Mars, women are from Venus.

John Gray

Addendumb: And dogs are from Pluto, donkeys from Uranus.

There are three kinds of men:
The ones who learn by reading.
The few who learn by observation.
The rest who have to pee on the electric fence and find out for themselves.

Will Rogers

Man is something like a sausage,
Very smooth upon the skin;
But you can never tell exactly
How much hog there is within.

MENTAL IMBALANCE
…mentally ill-arious.

One out of four people in this country is mentally imbalanced.
Think of your three closest friends. If they seem okay, then you're the one.

Ann Landers

You'll never have to twist my wrist
To get me to my analyst.
I love to talk, and so get rid
Of thoughts I've hidden since a kid.
Then I can look at what I did
And blame it all upon my id!

Herb Sufrin

MICROBES
Adam
Had 'em.

Stickland Gillilan

The microbe is so very small
You cannot make him out at all,
But many sanguine people hope
To see him through a microscope.
His jointed tongue that lies beneath
A hundred curious rows of teeth;
His seven tufted tails with lots
Of lovely pink and purple spots,
One each of which a pattern stands,
Composed of forty separate bands;
His eyebrows of a tender green;
All these have never yet been seen.
But scientists who ought to know,
Assure us that it must be so...
Oh, let us never, never doubt
What nobody is sure about.

Hilaire Belloc
The Microbe
1870-1953

MIDDLE AGE
...when everything starts to wear out, fall out, or spread out.

Every man is a fool or a physician at forty.
Thomas Fuller M.D.

It's when you're too young for Medicare and too old for women to care.

The five B's of middle age:
Baldness, bridgework, bifocals, bunions and bay windows.

Midlife crisis is what happens when you climb to the top of the ladder
and discover that it's against the wrong wall.
Joseph Campbell

Middle-age spread is the destiny that ends our shapes.

Adulteration: a person who has stopped growing at both ends and is now
growing in the middle.

Middle age is so much more
Than wrinkles on our faces;
It's when broad minds and narrow waists
Begin exchanging faces.

Charles Ghigna

MONEY
…still the most efficient labor saving device.

Franklin P. Jones

Two can live as cheaply as one, but only for half as long.

Inflation hasn't ruined everything. A dime can still be used as a screwdriver.

Designer jeans are priced so high. If I spend a hundred dollars for a pair of jeans, I expect a woman to be in them.

I had plastic surgery last week. I cut up my credit cards.

Henny Youngman

The business tycoon's daughter was on vacation from college and he was showing her around the newly acquired family estate. They stopped at the oversized swimming pool to watch several athletic and handsome young men perform from the diving board.
"Oh, Daddy!" exclaimed the daughter. "You've stocked it for me!"

The economy is so bad, if the bank returns your check marked, "Insufficient Funds," you call and ask them if they meant you or them.

I'm Rich!
Silver in the hair,
Gold in the teeth,
Crystals in the kidneys,
Sugar in the blood,
Lead in the butt,
Iron in the arteries,
And an inexhaustible supply of natural gas.
I never thought I'd accumulate such wealth.

MUSICAL THERAPY
If something is not worth saying, people sing it.

Johann Sebastian Bach wrote a great many compositions and had a large number of children. In between he practiced on the old spinster which he kept in his attic.

What do you get when you play country music backwards?
You get your wife back, your dog back, your car back.

My friend was trying to write a drinking song, but he couldn't get past the first few bars.

Song titles of note:
In the Still of the Night...... "Well, I'll drink to that."
Rap City Blue (With apologies to Gershwin).
I Ain't Never Gone to Bed With Ugly Women, But I Sure Woke Up With a Few.
Get Off The Gas Stove Granny, You're Too Old To Ride The Range.

The song with the longest title is:
"I'm a Cranky Old Yank in a Cranky Old Tank on the Streets of Yokohama with My Honolulu Mama Doin' Those Beat-o, Beat-o, Flat-on-My-Seat-o, Hirohito Blues."

Hoagy Carmichael

Memorable lyrics: How many roads must a man travel down before he admits he is lost?

You just sorta, smashed my aorta, then you stomped on my heart and smashed that sucker flat.

I know only two tunes: one of them is "Yankee Doodle" and the other isn't.

Ulysses S. Grant

Addendumb: It's "Dandy."

The Rolling Stones are on tour again. They were gonna call the tour "Concert or Your Money Back."

David Letterman

PS: At the least they're "gathering no moss."

Doctor, hurry, won't you hurry up and stop my worry,
Can't you see that I'm all a-flurry,
I've been troubled with ailment greatly, here lately.
Headache fixer, oh, you wonderful prescription fixer,
Won't you tell me why my shoulders keep going in the air?

Irving Berlin, 1913
They've Got Me Doing It Now.

"Irving, this is not one of your best, but I like it."

NAUSEATE
...inedible.

On a New York subway train, you get heavily fined if you spit.
On the other hand, you're allowed to throw up for nothing.
Lewis Grizzard

Upchucking: biofeedback.

Seasickness: Crossing the ocean by rail.

Vodka is tasteless going down, but it is memorable coming up.
Garrison Keillor

NEUROTIC
...a person in a clash by himself.

Al Bernstein

A person who worries about things that didn't happen in the past,
instead of worrying about something that won't happen in the future,
like normal people.

Reader's Digest

A neurotic is a man who builds a castle in the air. A psychotic is a man
who lives in it. And the psychiatrist is the man who collects the rent.
Robert Webb-Johnson

Neurotic means he is not as sensible as I am, and psychotic means
he's even worse than my brother-in-law.
Karl Menninger, M.D.

As soon as the rush is over, I'm going to have a nervous breakdown.
I worked for it. I owe it to myself, and nobody's going to deprive me of it.
Pearl Bailey

Neurologist: a super-charged electrician without the warranty.

Why Worry?
There are only two things to worry about:
Either you are well or you are sick.
If you are well, there's nothing to worry about.
But if you are sick,
There are only two things to worry about:
Either you get well or you die.

If you get well, there's nothing to worry about.
But if you die, there are only two things to worry about:
Either you will go to heaven or hell.
If you go to heaven, there's nothing to worry about.
But if you go to hell
You'll be so busy shaking hands with friends
You won't have time to worry.

NEUROPHARMACOLOGY
A new age for personality:

Are you satisfied with you? Who you are?
Does your id run amok among the odd?
Do you prefer type A or B or Z?
Just remember, a new day is dawning,
The age of neuropharmacology,
Where designer drugs drive us snug to treat
Pychoneuroimmonologic bugs.
Nevermore stressed, depressed or obsessed,
Living one's life in perpetual jest,
Exhilarated in new blessedness.

N.H.

NICOTINES
...the dangerous years.

Nicotine Patches: One man hated them saying, "First, they were hard to light. Then they didn't last very long."
     The doctor said, "Why not try putting them over your mouth?"

NITROUS OXIDE
...the only gas that's guaranteed to make you laugh.
Addendumb: If your dentist is out of laughing gas, tell him to begin with his best joke.

Professor: Give the most important fact about nitrates.
Student: They're cheaper than day rates.

NOISE
...earitation.

"Grandma, you have a suppository stuck in your ear."
"Oh, Thanks. I wondered what happened to my hearing aid."

After listening to Tallulah Bankhead struggle through a song, Jimmy
Durante confided, "I think you ought to have your tonsils out."
    She answered, "I've already had them out."
    Durante replied, "Then put them back in."

Your wife is at the front door yelling and your dog is at the back door
barking. Which do you let in first? The dog. When you let him in, he will
shut up.

I bought a wooden whistle, but it wooden whistle.
I bought a steel whistle, but it steel wooden whistle.
So I bought a tin whistle.
Now I tin whistle.

NONSENSE
...the objections made against this therapeutic text.
                         N.H.

Forgive me my nonsense as I forgive the nonsense of those who think they
talk sense.
                         Robert Frost

I like nonsense; it wakes up the brain cells.
                         Dr. Seuss

I am a nobody,
Nobody is perfect.
Therefore I am perfect.

NOSTALGIA
...a pain in the nose.

Romantics say "it's not what it used to be."

Instinct is the nose of the mind.
                      Delphine de Girardin

Chico Marx was once embarrassed upon hearing someone say, "Eureka."
Chico shot back, "You doan smella so good yourself."

Cyrano de Bergerac's nose:
Obvious: Excuse me, is that your nose, or did a bus park on your face?
Meteorological: Everybody take cover! She's going to blow!
Fashionable: You could de-emphasize your nose if you wore something
               larger, like Wyoming.
Personal: Well, here we are, just the three of us.
Laugh and the world laughs with you. Sneeze and it's 'Goodbye Seattle.'
Dirty: Your name wouldn't be Dick, would it?

Steve Martin
Roxanne

Ode to a Nose:
A bouquet of noses,
We didn't say roses,
Though roses are beautiful and sweet.
Tis the nose that tells us,
Enchants us, compels us
To scents good enough to eat.

NOVELTY

I can't understand why a person will take a year to write a novel when he
can buy one for a few dollars.

Fred Allen

My sole literary ambition is to write one good novel, then retire to my
hut in the desert, assume the lotus position, compose my mind and senses,
and sink into meditation, contemplating my novel.

Edward Abbey

From the moment I picked up your book until I laid it down,
I was convulsed with laughter. Some day I intend reading it.

Groucho Marx

NUDISTS

… persons who grin, bare, and share it.

I saw one bather at a nude beach seventy years old! And she was proud of it.
    She said, "What do you think of my birthday suit?"
    I said, "It needs ironing."

The proprietor of an art gallery in London showed art to a customer who
didn't know what he liked. He was shown a landscape, a still life, a portrait
and a floral piece. "Would you be interested in a nude?" he finally asked.

"Good heavens! No. I'm a physician."
English Digest

At our local nudist camp, a costume party was the highlight of the season. A lady with varicose veins won first prize by going as a road map.

A bather whose clothing was strewed
By breezes that left her quite nude,
Saw a man come along
And, unless I'm quite wrong,
You expected this line to be lewd.

NURSE
...one of the few who can tell you to drop your drawers without getting arrested.
Leslie Gibson, R.N.

Sign in emergency ward:
Interns think of God
Residents pray to God
Doctors believe they are God
Nurses are God.

War(d) words: "Would you like to speak to the doctor in charge or to the nurse who knows what's going on."

Nursery: a school for young nurses.

To Head Nurse: "Your title is amazing. I never knew nurses were so specialized."

Other Nurse Types:
RN — real nurse
LPN — let's play nurse
Petite — too cute for wards

One nurse was showing a young female graduate around the hospital. Stopping at the men's convalescent ward, she remarked "This ward is really dangerous. The patients are almost well."

Hugh Hefner now has 7 girlfriends — one for each day of the week. Someone needs to tell him that those are nurses.
Jay Leno

NURSING
...a hospital of hootenannies.

I majored in nursing. I had to drop it. I ran out of milk.
Judy Tenuta

Three reasons for breast-feedings:
The milk is always at the right temperature.
It comes in attractive containers.
The cat can't get it.
Irena Chalmeers

Nursing Homes: Be nice to your children. After all, they are going to choose your nursing home.
Steven Wright

NUTRITION
Let your food be your medicine and let your medicine be your food.
Hippocrates

Eat what you want and let the food fight it out inside.
Mark Twain

I'm president of the United States, and I'm not going to eat any more broccoli.
George H. Walker Bush

High-fiber makes you feel like a bran-new person.
Shelly Friedman

The four basic food groups: Fresh, Frozen, Fast and Junk.

An observant old codger named Browder
Said, "Now, between bean soup and chowder,
You'll find, my good friend,
That bean soup — in the end,
Will prove to be several times louder."

OBESITY
...circumferencely challenged.

It's surplus gone to waist.

The older you get, the tougher it is to lose weight.
By then your body and your fat are really good friends.

I would gladly lose weight but would hate it when people say,
"You're only half the man you used to be."

Shakespeare on Obesity: Whatever Romeo refused, Juliet.

Astringent: A thin man.

She weighed three hundred pounds.
Fat and high sugars were killing her I thought.
So, I thought.
I gave her a puppy with dark curly hair;
Nothing else had worked.
Walking the dog twice a day, I thought
Might persuade, might motivate.
She was pleased with my prescription,
She laughed, she rocked from side to side.
She lived for twelve years
Hugging that little black dog
While her lean husband
Walked it faithfully, twice a day.

John L. Wright M.D.
Walking the Dog

OBSTETRICS
When the doctor asked me if I wanted a bikini-cut for my C-section,
I said, "No. A bikini and a wine cooler is why I'm laying here now."

Kim Tavares

Menopause: The silence after a woman tells a man she is pregnant.

H. C. Wolford

Pregnancy is amazing! To think that you can create a human being just
with things you have around the house.

Amy Foster

OLD
...geriatrically gifted.

People of 70 you should not keep overnight, and do not invite a person of
80 to sit down.

Chinese Proverb

There are three ages of man: youth, middle age, and "Gee, you look good."
                                        Red Skelton

Old is when your wife says, "Let's go upstairs and make love," and you say,
"Honey, I can't do both."
                                        Red Buttons
Addendumb: Always know your vertigo.

Sign in store: NO SENIOR DISCOUNTS
            You have lived long enough to have saved money.

A senior citizen said to his eighty-year old buddy:
'So I hear you're getting married?'
'Yep!'
'Do I know her?'
'Nope!'
'This woman, is she good looking?'
'Not really'
'Is she a good cook?'
'Naw, she can't cook too well.'
'Does she have lots of money?'
'Nope, poor as a church mouse.'
'Why in the world do you want to marry her then?'
'Because she can still drive!'

As you age remember this,
Always follow your bliss
With wine, wood, books and friends.
Old wine is best to drink,
Old wood is best to burn,
Old authors best to read,
And old friends best to love,
If you run out of the above.

OPTIMIST
...an eye specialist.

Show me an optimist, and I'll show you a happy-condriac.

Some people are pessimistical optimists:
"Since the house is on fire, let us warm ourselves."

Never look backwards or you'll fall down the stairs.
Addendumb: Down with those people who are up all the time.

Optimist: "Good Morning, God."
Pessimist: "Good God! Morning!"

OPTOMETRISTS
...those who love to make spectacles of themselves.

Yesterday I was walking down the street wearing my glasses,
when all of a sudden my prescription ran out.

Steven Wright

Sign in Optometrist's office:
If You Don't See What You're Looking For,
You've Come To the Right Place.

I would have been an optometrist
But my professor and I
Did not see eye to eye.

ORGAN DONATION
…especially nice for the musically gifted.

When reviewing my driver's license at the age of 83 I was asked if I would
like to be an organ donor.
    I said, "Who would want them?"

Constance Dean

What do you call a cyclist who doesn't wear a helmet?
An organ donor.

David Perry

When our organs have been transplanted
And the new ones made happy to lodge in us,
Let us pray one wish be granted —
We retain our zones erogenous.

E.Y. Harburg
Seated One Day at the Organ

ORTHODONTIST
…one who invites you to put your money where your mouth is.

They like to brace the kids and strap the parents.

A lot of people have the reputation for being cheerful
when they're really just proud of their teeth.

OTOLARYNGOLOGIST
Posted sign: Specializing in ear, nose and throat.
Entrance in rear.

Strep Throat: hoarse and buggy.

Stethoscope: a magnifying glass for looking into peoples' chests with the ears.
                                              Leonard Lewis Levinson

He said my bronchial tubes were entrancing,
My epiglottis filled him with glee,
He simply loved my larynx,
But he never said he loved me.
                                              Cole Porter
                                              The Physician

OVATION
...a birth response to tremendous applause.

The doctor took my baby out of my wife's belly. Then he turned to me and
asked, "Mr. Goldthwait, would you like to cut the cord?"
    I answered, "Isn't there anyone more qualified?"

I was so ugly when I was born, the doctor slapped my mother.
                                              Henny Youngman

Helen: I'm going to have triplets.
Blanche: Congratulations.
Helen: My doctor tells me that triplets happen once every three million times.
Blanche: My God, Helen. When did you find the time to do the housework?

PACYDERMATOLOGIST
...an elephant skin doctor.

Last night I shot an elephant in my pajamas.
What he was doing in my pajamas, I'll never know.
                                              Groucho Marx

I have a face like an elephant's behind.

Charles Laughton
English actor

"I get it Charles. Bigger is not always better. I'm glad you don't have Elephantiasis."

Elephant stew recipe:
First shoot an elephant. This will yield about 3,500 pounds of fine meat. Add 100 pounds of salt. Sprinkle with pepper (enough to make the elephant sneeze). Assemble 10,000 gallons of water, one truckload of mixed vegetables and add two rabbits for flavoring. Now cut elephant meat into small pieces. (This takes about two months). Boil in covered swimming pool for two weeks. Add vegetables and rabbits. Simmer at 485. Remember, if adding rabbit, that not everyone likes hare in his stew. Serves about 7,350 people.

Patricia Foley Hinnen

He thought he saw an elephant,
That practiced on a fife:
He looked again, and found it was
A letter from his wife.
"At length I realize," he said,
"The bitterness of life."

Lewis Carroll

PAIN
... is deeper than all thought, laughter is higher than all pain.

Elbert Hubbard

When a pain is great enough, we will let anyone be doctor.

Mignon McLaughlin

My Nan was complaining of chest pains.
I said, "Are you all right, Nan?"
She said, "I think I've got vagina."

Peter Kay

"A strange click-clack in the back of your sacroiliac."

Harold Rome
South America, Take It Away

The pain-relieving ingredient, there's always got to be a lot of that. Nobody wants anything less than Extra-Strength. "Give me the maximum allowable human dosage. Figure out what will kill me, and then back it off a little bit."

Jerry Seinfeld

There was a faith healer of zeal
Who said, "Although pain isn't real,
If I sit on a pin
And it punctures my skin,
I dislike what fancy I feel."

PANACEA
Step up. Step right this way. Don't drag your feet.
Don't doubt, waver, or hesitate one bit.
Don't have to say to yourself, down the road,
When your wife, some night, kicks you out of bed
To sleep in the den — don't have to say then:
"Doctor Panacea could have helped me."
Folks, right here in my hand, in this small box,
Is *The Wonder Drug* — the miracle that
Cures depression, overweight, and back pains:
Try Acetyl-chlor-oxy-minophen.

Ken Bell

PARANOIA
The whole world isn't out to get you.
There are millions out there who don't care one way or another.

Tom Wilson
Ziggy

Even a paranoid can have enemies.

Henry Kissinger

Whenever you see two psychiatrists, don't let that paranoia.

Pronoia: a suspicion that people plot to make you happy.

PATHOLOGY
...the science of road building.

Psychopathic: taking the wrong fork in the road.

Psychopath: a laboratory physician analyzed.

Doctors are whippersnappers in iron white coats,
Who spy up your rectums and look down your throats,
And press you and poke you with sterilized tools,
And stab at solutions that pacify fools.
I used to revere them and do what they said,
'Til I learned what they learned on was already dead.

Gilda Radner

PATIENT
...an innocent person who is strip-searched and sentenced to a hospital
until the illness time is served or death has set in.

Jeff Charlebois
Medical Secrets Revealed

Patient compliance: Never take a pill that has more side effects than you
have symptoms.

Johnny Hart
B.C.

Out-patient: one who fainted.

Oral suspension: lack of patient counseling.

I know you have been waiting patiently for two hours,
that's why you're called the patient.

Some of my Patients (in 60 years of practice):

Esther Assalone	Kermit Longbottom
Flue Battle	Polyanna Miracle
Ova Bedford	Jacqueline Moneyham
Mary Bestfelt	Faith Mumchuck
Garland Butts	Alla Naibich
Lotta Cash	Allegra Nicodemus
Gaylord Valentine	Peter Pandelitis
Anita Crank	Blodwin Potee
Otto Filter	Tuesday Proffit
Joy Roach	Sylvester Ruebush
Precious Goodall	Maverich Ruff
Azalee Hagood	Fannie Rub
General Hardigree	Drucilla Schweinfus
Melody Hooker	Mao Ngoeun Sok
Olive Swearengin	Cast Steel Jr.
Claywymeica Lainhart	Mahlon Lemon

PEDICURE
…a well-baby clinic.

They solve the alimentary canal's loud voice on one end
and the lack of responsibility on the other end.

PENICILLIN
Prescriptions are preferable to surgery where the pen is mightier than the
sword.

The pen is also mightier than the sword,
if the sword is very small and the pen is real sharp.

Whoever said "the pen is mightier than the sword"
obviously never encountered automatic weapons.

General Douglas MacArthur

PERFUME
…body booze.

It's been called chemical warfare where both sides can win.

If I were a woman, I'd wear coffee as a perfume.

John Van Druten

When the soft air is sweet with the smell of lilacs, men often attribute it to
love, when they should attribute it to some drugstore.

The summer cologne was supposed to repel insects and attract men,
but they are still trying to get the bugs out of it.

A perfect pitch from a persistent perfume saleslady: "We are so sure of this
perfume that you can buy it now and let him pay later."

Much of it is made by the French
Who say, "It makes considerable scents
To spray it on negligees or negligents."

N.H.

PESSIMIST
…one who forgets to laugh, whereas an optimist laughs to forget.

The optimist sees the doughnut; the pessimist sees the hole.

McLandburgh Wilson

In my next life I would like to be a pessimist.
Then other people could spend all their time cheering me up.

Katherine Elizabeth Whitehorn

A pessimist feels bad when he feels good for fear he'll feel worse when he feels better.

PETS

A man is a dog's idea of what God should be.

Holbrook Jackson

Addendumb: And laughter is a human body wagging its tail.

Dogs come when they're called. Cats take a message and get back to you.

Mary Bly

My six year-old son just got a dog, so we're going to send him to obedience school. And if it works, we'll send the dog, too.

Outside of a dog, a book is man's best friend.
Inside of a dog, it's too dark to read.

Groucho Marx

Did you hear about the scientist who crossed a carrier pigeon with a woodpecker? He got a bird that not only delivers messages, but knocks on the door when it gets there.

John R. Fox

Asthma doesn't seem to bother me anymore unless I'm around cigars or dogs. The thing that would bother me the most would be a dog smoking a cigar.

Steve Allen

Bumper Sticker: My dog can lick your dog.
Addendumb: An elixir is what a dog does to his owner when she gives him a bone.

Phlebotomist: rectal spray for dogs.

When I was growing up, we had a petting zoo. We had two sections. There was a petting zoo and a heavy petting zoo, for people who really liked the animals a lot.

Ellen DeGeneres

I am fond of pigs. Dogs look up to us. Cats look down on us. Pigs treat us as equals.

Winston Churchill

PHARMACIST

...a pillar of society.
...a licensed drug pusher.
... a druggist who dispenses with accuracy.
... one who fills your pain.
...someone with a flare for medicine and business,
   good legs and an incredible bladder.
...Regulated pill healer. (R.Ph.)
...Rural pharmacist: One who is outstanding in his field.
...Elderly pharmacist: Not worth a dram when he loses all of his scruples.

Indispensable: a pharmacy consultant.

Pilliterate: a pharmacist unable to read a doctor's prescriptions.

Jeffrey & Carole Bloom

Addendumb: And an illiterate is one who can't read medical books.

A pharmacy intern wrote a book, but it was a drug on the market.

PHARMACOGNOCIST

...a crude druggist.

Some are called born-again plant worshippers. But few are chosen.

What is a weed? A plant whose virtues have not been discovered.

Ralph Waldo Emerson
1803-1882

If the hideous monster Frankenstein came face to face with the monster Marijuana, he would drop dead of fright.

Harry J. Anslinger
Commissioner of U.S. Bureau
of Narcotics from 1930 to 1962

PHILOSOPHY

...the microscope of thought.

Victor Hugo
1802-1885

My advice to you is to get married: if you find a good wife you'll be happy; if not, you'll become a philosopher.

Socrates

I have a simple philosophy. Fill what's empty. Empty what's full. Scratch where it itches.

Alice Roosevelt Longworth
1884-1980

I've developed a new philosophy. I only dread one day at a time.

Charles M. Schultz
Charlie Brown

PHLEGM
...an early form of humor.

What's the worst thing about having a heart-lung transplant?
You have to cough up somebody else's sputum.

Marti Murray, R.N.

He received from some thoughtful relations,
A spittoon with superb decorations.
When asked was he pleased,
He grimaced and wheezed,
"It's beyond all my expectorations."

PHYSICAL THERAPIST
...a person who uses pain and torture techniques to facilitate your healing process.

Jeff Charlebois

Masseuse: one who never rubs you the wrong way.

THE PILL
...a labor-saving device.

Last night I had a dream that all the babies prevented by the pill showed up. They were mad.

Steven Wright

Patient to pharmacist: "Why wouldn't I have birth control pills left over? I don't have sex every night?"

Pharmacist to patient: Take the pills three weeks on and one week off.
Patient: Tell that to my husband.

What is an oral contraceptive?
The word "No."

They've got a new birth control pill for men now. I think that's fair.
It makes a lot of sense to take the bullets out of the gun than to wear a
bulletproof vest.

Greg Travis

PILLAGE
…to plunder a pharmacy.

There's not a pill for every ill. Some prefer suppositories and other devices.

I used to scoff at poppa
For the many pills he popped.
Poppa's gone. Now I'm a popper, too.
And I'm gonna keep on poppin'
Like my Poppa 'til I drop!
I'd opt to stop but that would not
Be quite the proper thing to do.

Don Weill

PILL DRILL
Repeat after me…
This small white pill is what I munch
At breakfast and right after lunch.
I take the pill that's Kelly green
Before each meal and between.
These loganberry-colored pills
I take for early morning chills.
I take the pill with zebra stripes
To cure my early evening gripes.
These orange-tinted ones, of course,
I take to cure my charley horse.
I take three blues at half-past eight
To slow my exhalation rate.
On alternate nights at 9:00 P.M.
I swallow pinkies, four of them.
The reds, which make my eyebrows strong,
I eat like popcorn all day long.

The speckled browns are what I keep
Beside my bed to help me sleep.
This long flat one is what I take
If I should die before I wake.

Dr. Suess
You're Only Old Once

PLACEBO
...a hypochondriac's drug of choice.

Can placebos cause side effects? If so, are the side effects real?
George Carlin

Damital: a placebo that works.

After sending a parcel to European relatives during the war, we received a
very grateful letter with this paragraph:
    If you can, please send us more pills. We didn't know what they were
until Cousin Lempi came — she has studied English, you know — and
read the name for us. Then we gave them all to Uncle Paul, who has been
suffering from rheumatism and he feels much better now. He says it is the
best medicine he ever took. The pills are called "Life Savers."
Alice Murdock

PLASTIC SURGERY
..when beauty is nip and tuck.

She gets her looks from her father. He's a plastic surgeon.

I was going to have plastic surgery until I noticed that the doctor's office
was full of portraits by Picasso.
Rita Rudner

When the woman who had her face lifted saw the surgeon's bill, her face
fell down again.

One popular new plastic surgery technique is called lipografting, or fat
recycling, wherein fat cells are removed from one part of your body that is
too large, such as your buttocks, and injected into your lips. People will
then be literally "kissing your ass."
Dave Barry

Plastic surgeon: a surgeon who takes credit cards.

Due to some doctor's sloppy writing, instead of being taken to Detox, she was taken to Botox. She's still drinking and drugging herself like there's no tomorrow, but she looks fabulous.

PMS
...hormonally challenged.

It allows a woman, once a month, to act like men do every day.

My license plate says PMS. Nobody cuts me off.
Wendy Liebman

PMS jokes aren't funny; period.

PODIATRY
Great ache corns from little toe corns grow.

Dancing is podiatry in motion.
Addendumb: A chicken dancing is poultry in motion.

Until you've walked a mile in another man's shoes,
you have no idea how painful blisters can be.
Doug Kime
"But at least you have an extra pair of shoes!"

Callus: the agony of defeat.

In Extremis:
I saw my toes the other day.
I hadn't looked at them for months.
Indeed, they might have passed away.
And yet they were my best friends once.
When I was small, I knew them well.
I counted on them up to ten
And put them in my mouth to tell
The larger from the lesser. Then
I loves them better than my ears,
My elbows, adenoids, and heart.
But with the swelling of the years
We drifted toes and I apart.
Now gnarled and pale, each said j accuse! —
I hid them quickly in my shoes.
Bruce Lansky
Lighten Up

POLLEN
The Allergist's Lament (with apologies to Joyce Kilmer)

I used to think that I could see
A pollen lovely as a tree.
The sneezing, wheezing of the masses
Caught betwixt the leaves and grasses.
Unless the pollens start to fall,
I won't find any rest at all.

N.H.

POLYESTROUS
...horny animals.

A lady had two monkeys and was very fond of them. One of them took sick and died. Soon the other died of a broken heart. Wishing to keep them, the kindly lady took them to the taxidermist. The man asked her if she would like them mounted.

"Oh, no," she replied, "just have them holding hands."

A man seeking a hotel room for himself and his dog received the following reply from an innkeeper in Kingston, Jamaica:

"I've been in the hotel business for 40 years and never had to eject a disorderly dog. Never has a dog set fire to a bed. Never has he sneaked a girl into his room. Never has a dog stolen a towel or blanket or gotten drunk. Your dog is very welcome. If he will vouch for you, you can come along as well."

Parade

POTIONS (that stand the test of time)
Fillet of a fenny snake
In a cauldron boil and bake.
Eye of newt, and toe of frog;
Wool of bat, and tongue of dog;
Adders fork and blind-worms sting;
Lizards' legs and howlets' wing —

William Shakespeare
Macbeth

Beware of the stir-crazy druggist with a caldron in the back.

The pellet with the poison is in the vessel with the pestle. The chalice from the palace has the brew that is true.

Danny Kaye
The Court Jester

PRAYER

Forgive, O Lord, my little jokes on thee, and I'll forgive thy great big joke on me.

Robert Frost

Sam shows up at a revival meeting, seeking help. "I need you to pray for my hearing," he tells the preacher. The preacher put his fingers on Sam's ears and prays and prays. When he's done, he asks, "How's your hearing now?" Sam tells him, "I don't know. I don't go to court till next Tuesday."

James Hoskin

Dear God, My prayer for the New Year is for a fat bank account and a thin body. Please don't mix these up like you did last year. Amen.

May those that love us, love us.
And those that don't love us,
May God turn their hearts,
And if He doesn't turn their hearts,
May He turn their ankles
So we'll know them by their limping.

Old Irish Prayer

PREGNANCY

Having a baby is like taking your lower lip and forcing it over your head.

Carol Burnett

Why does it take millions of sperm to fertilize one female egg?
Because they won't ask for directions.

A man speaks frantically into the phone. "My wife is pregnant, and her contractions are only two minutes apart."
    The doctor asks, "Is this her first child?"
    The man shouts "No, you idiot, this is her husband."

Labor pains: previews of coming attractions.

Sing a song of Clomid
A pelvis full of dye.
Four and twenty studies
Your HMO won't buy.
When the tests are finished,
The docs and nurses sing,
"By the time we get you pregnant,
You won't own a thing."

Howard Bennett, M.D.

PRESCRIPTION
...hieroglyphics written by a physician and translated by a pharmacist into dollar signs.

P.S. on Rx: "I got mine. Now you get yours."

PRESCRIPTION DIRECTIONS
q.i.d. is a Latin term. It means, "There's no way I'm taking this pill four times daily."
Ryan James, M.D.

Before giving my mother the medicine that I had picked up at our neighborhood pharmacy, I read the label: "Take one teaspoonful at breakfast and suffer."
Sam Herman

Place three drops in left eye every two hours while awake for five days.

Nystatin Vaginal Suppositories, #24, Sig:
Insert one daily in vagina until exhausted.

Rx Consultation: "How effective are these pills?" a patient asked the pharmacist.
   "Well, some anti-depressants are far more effective when taken with lots of water gently rolling off an ocean shore while dreaming of paradise. Soon you'll find yourself flinging those pills way out into the deep."

PROCRASTINATION
We'll get to this one later.

PROCTOLOGIST
...an analyst.
...a doctor who can't remember faces but always stands behind his work.

Sign on proctologist's door: To expedite your visit, please back in.

Why are hemorrhoids called hemorrhoids and asteroids called asteroids?
Wouldn't it be better if it was the other way around?
But if that was true, then a proctologist would be a astronaut.
Robert Schimmel

Proctologists never consider hindsight a source of embarrassment.

Proctology: Holistic therapy.

Names mean everything. A psychiatrist and a proctologist decided
to cut expenses to start their practices in the same office building. They
brainstormed over what to call themselves "Minds and Behinds" would
not do. "Hysterias and Posteriors?" Not good. Then one said "How about
The Hokey Pokey Clinic and A Place To Turn Yourself Around?" After
a good laugh, they decided to call themselves "Odds And Ends."

PROCTOSCOPE
...a super-dooper pooper snooper.

Many look at the proctoscope as a rearview mirror and the endoscope as
the last look.

People in the media say they must look at the president with a microscope.
I don't mind a microscope, but boy, when they use a proctoscope,
that's going too far.

Richard M. Nixon

PROSIT
...a Teutonic anti-depressant.

In heaven I am told, "There is no beer."
All the more reason to drink it here.

Slam Dunk (With apologies to Dr. Seuss)
I would drink beer with a goat on a boat,
In a box in my socks,
In a car, at a bar,
I do, I do, I do like beer!!
Slammed I am.

PROZAC (Fluoxetine)
T oday we have a new designer drug.
R elief from the blues it will guarantee.
Y ou won't know how good it feels 'til you're well.
A pril showers leave; then may June arrive.
P ut your cares away for good; start smiling.
R epeat the dose, and it's better each time.
O verall there will be nothing but gain.
Z est and zeal replace the awful doldrums.
A ll the benefit without the side effects.
C hasing the mood, it leaves us dry and high.

Al Corsbie

PSYCHEDELI
...where people eat healthy foods they don't like.

Older people shouldn't eat healthy foods. They need all the preservatives they can get.

Robert Orben

As for butter versus margarine, I trust cows more than chemists.

Joan Gussow

Psychedelirium Tremens:
Remember when HIPPIE meant big in the hips,
And a TRIP involved travel in ships?
POT was a pan for cooking things in,
And HOOKED was how the rug might have been?
When lights, not people were turned ON and OFF,
And THE PILL might be for a cough?
SQUARE meant a 90-degree angled form,
And COOL was a temperature not quite warm?
ROLL was a bun, ROCK was a stone,
And HANG-UP was the thing you did to a phone?
When SWINGER was one you swung in a swing,
And PAD was a soft cushiony thing?
Words once sensible and serious
Are making the FREAK SCENE PSYCHEDELIRIOUS.
It's GROOVY MAN, but English it's not.
Me thinks the language has gone to POT.

PSYCHIATRIST
...a doctor who doesn't have to worry as long as other people do.

It's the next man you start talking to after you start talking to yourself.

Fred Allen

Anybody who goes to a psychiatrist ought to have their head examined.

Samuel Goldwyn

He is always called a nerve specialist because it sounds better, but everyone knows he's sort of a janitor in a looney bin.

P.G. Wodehouse
1881-1975

Are you a psychiatrist?
Why do you ask?
You are a psychiatrist.

Psychiatrist to nurse: "Just say we're very busy. Don't say, It's a madhouse!"

I told my wife I was seeing a psychiatrist. Then she told me the truth.
She was seeing a psychiatrist, two plumbers and a bartender.
Rodney Dangerfield

Socialized medicine: when the psychiatrist lies down on the couch with you.

I went to my psychiatrist to be psychoanalyzed,
To find out why I killed the cat and blackened my wife's eyes.
He laid me on a downy couch to see what he could find,
And this is what he dregged up from my subconscious mind.
When I was one, my mommy locked my dolly in the trunk,
And so it follows naturally that I am always drunk.
When I was two, I saw my father kiss the maid one day.
That is why I suffer now from kleptoman-e-ay.
When I was three, I suffered from ambivalence toward my brothers.
That is just the reason why I poisoned all my lovers.
I'm so glad since I have learned that lesson so well taught,
That everything I do that's wrong is someone else's fault.
John Guest
Guilt, Responsibility

PSYCHOLOGIST
...a bartender who hates to see a grown man dry.
N.H.

It's a man you pay to ask questions your wife asks you for nothing.

Someone you go to when you're slightly cracked,
And continue attending until you're totally broke.
Tony Hancock

Feminine psychology: Smart enough to ask your husband's advice
but not being dumb enough to take it.

PSYCHOTIC
You've no idea what a poor opinion I have of myself
and how little I deserve it.

Basically my wife was immature.
I'd be in my bath, and she'd come in and sink my boats.
Woody Allen

Psychophobia: The compulsion when using a host's bathroom, to peer behind the shower curtain and make sure no one is waiting for you.

Rich Hall

Two psychiatry patients were discussing their conditions:
Said the first, "I'd be fine if I didn't have this gaping hole in my head."
Replied the second,"You're lucky. I have two gaping holes in my head."
Retorted the first, "I'm so sick of your 'holier–than-thou'attitude."

PUBERTY
The cause of changing the voice at the years of puberty seemeth to be, for that when much of the moisture of the body, which did before irrigate the parts, is drawn down to spermatical vessels, it leaveth the body more hot than it was, whence cometh the dilation of the pipes.

Francis Bacon
1561-1626

Addendumb: The pub is where Bacon learned about puberty.

QUADRUPLE BYPASS
...the ramp you missed four exits back.

Johnny Hart
B.C.

The "O" turn — a new female driving maneuver, during which they start a "U" turn and then change their minds.

Royal Neighbor

Two wrongs don't make a right, but three left turns do.

QUININE
...the bark that is better than its bite.

Much are we beholden to physicians, who only prescribe the bark of the quinquina, when they might oblige their patients to swallow the whole tree.

Sir David Dalrymple
Lord Hailes, 1797

If her lips are on fire and she trembles in your arms, forget her.
She's got malaria.

Jackie Kannon

RABIES
Every man gets mad when a dog bites him, whether the dog is mad or not.

The noblest of all dogs is the hot dog; it feeds the hand that bites it.
> Laurence J. Peter

Rabid Fan: a drunk in a ball park.

RADIOLOGIST
…X-rated.

It's a doctor who sees right through you.

The doctor X-rayed my head and found nothing.
> Dizzy Dean

RECTALGIA
…a pain in the rear, mostly evident in others.

Who invented the brush they put next to the toilet? That thing hurts.
> Andy Andrews

"Rectum?"
"No, it damn near killed him."

A doctor about ready to write a prescription reaches into his inside coat pocket and pulls out a rectal thermometer. He looks at it a moment, then comments, "Some asshole's got my pen."
> Benjamin Felson, M.D.

RELIGION
Life is God's joke on us. It's our mission to figure out the punch line.
> John Guarrine

In Edmonton, Canada a church had a large sign outside: JESUS SAVES. Across the street from the church was a large supermarket with a sign: BUT WE SAVE YOU MORE.
> Sister Mary Christelle Macaluso
> *The Fun Nun*

I wonder what our ancestors would think of our country today?
When I get to heaven, I'll ask them.
What if they didn't go to heaven?
Then you ask them.

An elderly man walks into a confessional. "Father, I'm a ninety-five-year-old widower, I have many children and grandchildren, and yesterday I went out on a date with a twenty-five-year-old supermodel!"

The priest says, "Well, that doesn't sound like a sin. You should know that as a Catholic. Dating is not a sin."

The penitent answers, "Oh, I'm not a Catholic, Father. I'm Jewish."

The priest says, "So why are you telling me all this?"

"I'm ninety-five years old! I'm telling everybody!"

Fr. James Martin S.J.

Life for some is to sow wild oats during the week and then go to church on Sunday and pray for a crop failure.

Church bulletin bloopers: Remember in prayer the many who are sick of our community.

Smile at someone who is hard to love.
Say "Hell" to someone who doesn't care much about you.

The senior choir invites all the members of the congregation who enjoy sinning to join us.

Closing sermon:
Why should the Devil get all the good tunes,
The booze and the neon and Saturday night,
The swaying in darkness, the lovers like spoons?
Why should the Devil get all the good tunes?
Does he hum them to while away sad afternoons
And the long, lonesome Sundays? Or sing them for spite?
Why should the Devil get all the good tunes,
The booze and the neon and Saturday night?

REMEDY
When a lot of remedies are suggested for a disease, that means it can't be cured.
Anton Chekov M.D.
1860-1904

For bags: A cure for bags under the eyes is to sleep upside down.
The bags often work through a less noticeable part of the body.
Mary Dunn

For laryngitis: Try listening for a change.

For wrinkled skin: More than likely your navel has come untied.
Gather the folds of the skin at your navel and tie them around a short
stick. Twist the stick until your upper lip is drawn up into a sneer, then
back off a turn and a half. This should remove most of the wrinkles.
Do not let go of the stick without a crash helmet.

Lockjaw: A great halitosis remedy.

Nosebleed: The best way to avoid it is to keep out of other people's business.

The root elixirs I've devoured,
Those tonics brewed from barks of trees,
My taste for secret mixtures soured
A twinge, a hurt, a feeling faint
I now ignore, you see:
'Cause patent medicines just ain't
What they're quacked up to be.

                                        Herb Sufrin

RESTAURANT
The other night I ate at a real nice family restaurant.
Every table had an argument going.

                                        George Carlin

The food here is terrible, and the portions are too small.

                                        Woody Allen

Diner: What's the specialty of the house?
Waiter: The Heimlich maneuver.

Sadie, I — I tink I svallowed a bone.
Are you choking, Hyman?
No, I'm serious!

Tokyo hotel menu: All vegetables in this restaurant are washed in water
passed by our head chef.

Sign in restaurant window: Wanted — man to wash dishes and two
waitresses.

A diner while dining at Crewe
Found a rather large mouse in his stew.
Said the waiter, "Don't shout
And wave it about,
Or the rest will be wantin one too,"

RETINITIS PIGMENTOSA
...a potent Mexican concoction that makes fat guys see double and get up to dance.

It was one tequila, two tequila, three tequila, floor!
                                                    Dennis Miller

RETIREMENT
I am retired. I was tired yesterday and I'm tired again today.

Retirement means twice as much husband and half as much money.

At retirement party: "We can't give you a gold watch, but feel free to call us whenever you want to know what time it is."

ROSACEA
Until cured, I don't have to wear my red clown nose.

A red-nosed man may not be a drinker, but he will find nobody to believe it.

I had a rose named after me and I was very flattered. But I was not pleased to read the description in the catalogue: "No good in a bed, but fine against a wall."
                                                    Eleanor Roosevelt

SALIVA
Does the name Pavlov ring a bell?

Secretion: Not being truthful with your doctor.

Why do we know so little about the salivary glands?
It's because they are so secretive.

SCHIZOPHRENIA

...a state in which two can live as cheaply as one.

Robert Williams

I always wanted to be someone, but I should have been more specific.

Lily Tomlin

Addendumb: Be yourself. Everyone else is taken.

Schizo Post Cards:
Having a wonderful time. Wish I were here.
Having a wonderful time. Wish you were her.
Having a wonderful time. Wish I could afford it.

Neurosis are red,
Depression is blue.
I'm schizophrenic.
How about you?

SCHOOL

Methylphenidate (Ritalin): Each morning we begin our school day with a minute of silent medication.

When I was in school, there was no Ritalin for attention deficit disorder, just a big nun with a ruler.

Maureen Dowd

There was a time when I hated school. I didn't want to go. My parents asked me why? I said, "The teachers hate me, the students hate me. The janitor hates me. I won't go." But they insisted. "You must go, you're the principal."

Sex education in school may be a good idea, but there should be no homework.

Bill Cosby

Old teachers never die, they just lose their principals.
Old principals never die, they just lose their faculties.
Old students never die, they just lose their class.

SENILITY

...the wit of longevity.

R. W. Jackson

"Don't worry about senility," my grandfather used to say.
"When it hits you, you won't know it."

Bill Cosby

At a senior home, a big time celebrity asked a resident, "Do you know who I am?"

"No, but if you go to the front desk, they will tell you."

Prayer:
God, grant me the senility to forget the people I never liked anyway,
The good fortune to run into the ones I do,
And the eyesight to tell the difference.

SEX
…the biggest nothing of all time.

Andy Warhol

It' a misdemeanor. The less you have, de meanor you get.

Charles Pierce

Sex today is big business. Some people can remember when it was just a maw and paw operation.

"I don't see much of Alfred anymore since he got interested in sex."

Mrs. Alfred Kinsey

The sexual revolution is over and the microbes won.

P. J. O'Rourke
Give War a Chance

There will always be the battle of the sexes,
because men and women want different things.
Men want women and women want men.

SEXAGENARIAN
…a sexually-focused chronological gifted individual.

Robert B. Moore

At 60 you still get the urge but can't remember what for exactly.

A man is as old as the woman he feels.

Groucho Marx
Addendumb: Today a grouchy man is as old as the Viagra he feels.

131

An old man went to see his doctor for a checkup.

At the end of the visit the doctor said, "I think you should cut your sex life in half."

"Which half, talking about it or thinking about it?"

Doctors say you can enjoy sex way past eighty, but not as a participant.
                                                    Phyllis Diller

Sex after ninety is like trying to shoot pool with a rope.
                                                    George Burns

Safe sex for seniors: keep an oxygen tank at bedside along with a defibrillator.

I cannot see
I cannot pee
I cannot chew
I cannot screw
Oh, my God, what can I do?
My memory shrinks
My hearing stinks
No sense of smell
I look like hell
My mood is bad — can you tell?
My body's drooping
Have trouble pooping
The Golden Years have come at last
The Golden Years can kiss my ass.

                                                    Doctor Suess
                                                    The Cat in the Hat on Aging

SILICONES
...funny-looking bras for those who love to make mountains out of molehills.

I think Western Union should have a service where women with really big ones come to your house and sing *Happy Birthday.* They could call it a mammogram.

Never go to a plastic surgeon for silicone implants if he charges a flat fee.

Good cheekbones are the brassiere of old age.
                                                    Barbara de Portago

SITZ BATH
...poor man's spa.

I test my bath before I sit,
And I'm always moved to wonderment
That what chills the finger not a bit
Is so frigid upon the fundament.

Ogden Nash

SKELETON
...bare essentials.

It was so hot we took off all our skin and sat around in our bones.

Sign in graveyard: Due to the shortage of manpower, graves will be dug by our skeleton staff.

SKIN
...is like wax paper that holds everything in without dripping.
Art Linkletter

It's not wrinkles. I just have too much skin for the size of my face.
Barbara Colson

I'm tired of all this nonsense about beauty being skin deep.
That's enough. What do you want? An adorable pancreas?
Jean Kerr

Skin Care: I eat plenty of garlic and Limburger cheese.
Keeps people far away...which is where I look best.
Grampa (Abe) Simpson

Moles: God's punctuation marks.

Please scratch my back and I'll make you rich,
I can't reach the place I itch.
Oo-ee-ooo, that feels fine —
Thank you, friend, a million times.
Give you money? Why? What for?
I ain't itching anymore.

Shel Silverstein

SLEEP
A good laugh and a long sleep are the best cures.
Irish Proverb

Early to bed and early to rise, and you'll meet very few of our best people.
George Ade

Sometimes I wake up grumpy; other times I let him sleep.

You say you need your Z's. You can't sleep?
You've exhausted your pills. You're tired of counting sheep?
Ever wonder what doctors do for sleep?
They dream of their blessings, Sleeping Beauty and Little Bo Peep.
N.H.

SLEEPING PILL
I slept like a log last night.
Addendumb: I must have. I woke up in the fireplace.

Sleepwalking: a good way to get your rest and your exercise
at the same time.

My grandmother was a very tough woman. She buried three husbands.
Two of them were just napping.
Rita Rudner

Here's something that causes much weeping —
The nurse to your room comes creeping.
She gives you a shake,
And when you awake,
Makes you swallow a pill for sleeping.

SMILE
...simply a flip of a frown.

It's a face-lift that's in everyone's price range and the second best thing you can do with your lips.

Did you know that even a fake smile releases dopamine, adrenalin and serotonin? All are good brain drugs. You can't buy these at a drug store. Well, not easily anyway.

Some people are like Slinkies — not really good for anything, but you can't help smiling when you see one tumble down the stairs.

Always be ready to go the extra smile.

No matter how grouchy you're feeling,
You'll find the smile more or less healing.
It grows in a wreath
All around the front teeth,
Thus preserving the face from congealing.

Anthony Euwer

SMOKING
When I was young, I kissed my first woman and smoked my first cigarette
on the same day. Believe me, never have I wasted any more time on tobacco.

Arturo Toscanini
1867-1957

Smoking…kills you, and if you're killed, you've lost a very important part
of your life.

Brooke Shields

The only way to stop smoking is to just stop. No ifs, ands or butts.

Bumper sticker rebuttal: Harassing me about smoking may be hazardous
to your health.

Mr. Glubb puffed heavily on his cigar while loitering in a shopping mall
drugstore.
    The pharmacist said to him, "Please sir, there's no smoking in the store."
    "But I just bought the cigar here," Mr. Glubb said.
    "Look," the pharmacist said, "we sell laxatives and condoms here too,
but you can't enjoy them on the premises."

SNORING
…the sounds of silence.

Laugh and the world laughs with you. Snore and you sleep alone.

Anthony Burgess

He: I slept like a log.
She: More like a sawmill.

There was an old man of Calcutta,
Who coated his tonsils with butta,
Thus converting his snore
From a thunderous roar
To a soft, oleaginous mutta.

Ogden Nash

135

SORGHUM
...a dental problem.

"Your teeth are fine, but your gums have got to go."

Last week I noticed my gums were shrinking. Then I found out that I was brushing my teeth with Preparation H.

She laughs at everything you say. Why? Because she has fine teeth.
Benjamin Franklin

Always be true to your teeth or they will be false to you.

Your teeth, my love, are like the stars
That shine so bright above you.
Their pearly whiteness holds a charm
Which makes the whole world love you.
When e'er your eyes look into mine,
They set my pulses dancing,
But when you smile at me, my love,
'Tis then you're most entrancing.
Those lovely teeth — I'll sing their praise
As long as I am able.
But do you think it proper, love,
To leave them on the table?

SPEAKING
Public speaking is the art of making deep noises from the chest sound like important messages from the brain.

I know that you believe you understand what you think I said,
but I am not sure you realize that what you heard is not what I meant.
Berry & Homer Inc.

Speak softly and carry a big stick.
Theodore Roosevelt

It's useless to hold a person to anything he says while he's in love, drunk, or running for office.
Barack Obama

Edison did not invent the first talking machine. He invented the first one that could be turned off.

Blessed are they who have nothing to say,
and who cannot be persuaded to say it.

James Russell Lowell
1819-1891

Speaking is the number one thing that people fear the most. Fear of dying
is way down on the list. So, it is easier to be in the coffin at a funeral than
to give the eulogy.

Worst intro of all time: "Ladies and Gentlemen — the President of the
United States — Hoobert Herver."

Harry Von Zell, 1928
Inaugural Address

In Praise of a Successful Preacher:
We gave him twenty minutes.
He finished up in ten.
Oh, there's a prince of speakers
And a servant unto men!
His diction wasn't very much;
He hemmed and hawed a bit.
Still he spoke a lot of sense
And after that he quit.
At first we sat quite paralyzed,
Then cheered and cheered again.
We gave him twenty minutes,
And he finished up in ten.

St. Andrews Parish
London. England

SPECIALIST
..one who knows more and more about less and less.

William J. Mayo, M.D.
1861-1939

Multiple Specialists:
a rash of dermatologists
a hive of allergists
a scrub of interns
a chest of phthisiologists
a giggle of nurses
a flood of urologists
a pile of proctologists
an eyeful of opthalmologists

a whiff of anesthesiologists
a staff of bacteriologists
a cast of orthopedic rheumatologists
a gargle of laryngologists.

SPECIMEN
...an Italian astronaut.

An elderly woman went to the doctor's office with a beautiful butterfly mounted under glass and presented it to the nurse. The nurse said, "This is very nice, Mrs. Brown, but it's not the type of specimen we had in mind."

SPORTS
...the toy department of life.

Howard Cosell

A small college at an athletic meet had a cross-eyed javelin thrower.
He didn't win any metals but he sure kept the crowd alert.
Addendumb: Another javlander won the coin toss and chose to receive.

In the 1978 film *Grease*, a good line was delivered by Eve Arden in the role of the high school principal, Miss McGee: "If you can't be an athlete, be an athletic supporter."

A baseball broadcaster of the New York Yankees said, "(Dave) Winfield goes back to the wall, he hits his head on the wall and it rolls off! It's rolling all the way back to second base. This is a terrible thing for the Padres."

Jerry Coteman
On the Air

"See the New York Jets play the Cincinnati Bagels this Sunday on NBC."
Unknown TV announcer

Is golf a sport or a game?
Ask this of those who play in the rain.
The tart retort is a bit of a curse
Proving why golf is flog in reverse.

N.H.

STOOL (scatological)
Always look out for number one and be careful not to step in number two.
Rodney Dangerfield

It wasn't the canine who stoically stole in, stooled, and stole out again,
But it was the cat who cunningly crept in, crapped, and crept out again.

Klinker's pooper blooper: "What are you in jail for?"
"I'm in for armed robbery. Some dirty squeal pigeon stooled on me."

STRESSED
…is DESSERTS spelled backwards.

They have a great drug now. It doesn't make you relaxed. It just makes
you enjoy being tense. But, Jesus, when you don't have any money,
the problem is food. When you have enough money, it's sex. When you
have both, it's health. You worry about getting ruptured or something.
If everything is simply jake, then you're frightened to death.
                    V.P. Donleavy

I burned my candle at both ends,
And now have neither foes nor friends;
For all the lovely light begotten,
I'm paying now in feeling rotten.

                         Samuel Hoffenstein

SUICIDE
…a permanent solution to a temporary problem.
                         Phil Donahue

If I had no sense of humor, I should long ago have committed suicide.
                    Mahatma Gandhi

I was thinking about committing suicide, but I have a tendency to
procrastinate, so I kept putting it off. They say procrastination is a bad
thing, but it saved my life.
                         Shasi Bhatia

When you get to the end of your rope, tie a knot on it and hang on.
Then swing.
                         Leo Buscaglia

Sign in Cincinnati Health Department: If you're considering suicide,
it wouldn't kill you to call us first. 281-CARE

Razors pain you,
Rivers are damp,
Acids stain you
And drugs cause cramp.
Guns aren't lawful,
Nooses give,
Gas smells awful,
You might as well live.

Dorothy Parker

SUNBURN
...a fry in the ointment.

I never expected to see the day when girls would sunburn in the places
they do today.

Will Rogers

Tanning: a process of making leather.

All right, go lie upon the beach,
To bake beyond the water's reach;
But if you're blistered when you quit,
Remember that you basked for it.

Paul Flowers

SURGERY
Before undergoing a surgical operation, arrange your temporal affairs.
You may live.

Ambrose Bierce

Patient: Doc, I'm scared. This is my first operation.
Doctor: I know how you feel. This is my first operation.

I was real calm about the operation 'til I realized what I was doing.
I'm lying there naked on a table in front of people I don't know.
And they have knives. What's wrong with this picture?

Tom Parks

Did you hear about the guy whose whole left side was cut off?
He's all right now.

In ancient times health care professionals in tropical areas used large ants as sutures. Their jaws were strong and continued to grip even after death. When each ant bit, the caregiver capitated it. This gave rise to the practice of "Suture Self!"

SURGEON
...a plumber who works standing up.

A guy who tells you if you don't cut out something, he'll cut something out of you.

A stitch in time saves nine malpractice suits.

If a man still has his appendix, gall bladder, tonsils, thyroid, spleen, two kidneys and other assorted parts, ten to one he's a surgeon.

Naval Surgeons: Proof positive that medical specialization has gone too far.

As a surgeon, I prefer Shockley's scalpels. They are sharper, stronger, lighter. I prefer Shockley's scalpels for cutting out the appendix, the gall bladder, ulcers. Even for slicing pumpernickel. Shockleys will surprise you. Addendumb: It's the best thing since sliced bread.

Once I was sick and I had to go to an ear, nose, and throat man to get well. There are ear doctors, nose doctors, throat doctors, gynecologists, proctologists — any place you've got a hole, there's a guy who specializes in your hole. They make an entire career out of that hole. And if the ear doctor, nose doctor, throat doctor, gynecologist, or proctologist can't help you, he sends you to a surgeon. Why? So he can make a new hole.
                                        Alan Prophet

TATTOO
...body art to go.

Computers are everywhere. Now tattoo parlors have spell check.

On the chest of a barmaid in Sale
Were tattooed for prices of ale,
And on her behind,
For the sake of the blind,
Was the same information in Braille.

TEETOTALER
...a gift of the spirit.

I come from a family where gravy is considered a beverage.
Erma Bombeck

One reason why I don't drink is because I wish to know when I'm having a good time.
Nancy Astor

It's easy enough to be pleasant
And to sing of joy and good cheer;
But the man worthwhile
Is when the doctor cuts out his beer.

TELEVISION
...an electronic tranquilizer.

Before TV, no one knew what a headache looked like.

Sex on television can't hurt you unless you fall off.
Woody Allen

TV advertising: There are so many TV commercials now that what used to be a simple station break now sounds like a compound fracture.

"Tonight's program is sponsored by pills, Red pills, Blues pills, Green pills, Purple pills. Pills, pills and more pills! Ask your doctor if pills are right for you."
Funny Times

"My show is the stupidest show on TV. If you are watching it, get a life!"
Jerry Springer

My six-year-old grandson watches a lot of TV. This became apparent the day he asked his father, "Am I healthy enough for sexual activity?"
John Ball

We all have to go sometime. I usually go during the commercials.

From irate viewer to TV set: "Of course I'm bothered by an upset stomach, you idiot! It's your stupid commercial that upset my stomach."

TESTICLE
...a funny exam question.

The man who tickles himself can laugh when he chooses.
German Proverb

If quizzes are quizzical, what are tests?

TIME
...is an herb that cures all diseases.

Benjamin Franklin

Time wounds all heels.

Jane Ace

Addendumb: And time and a half heals them faster.

There is never enough time, unless you're serving it.

Malcolm Forbes

I have noticed that people who are late are often so much jollier than the people who have to wait for them.

E.V. Lucas

When a man sits with a pretty girl for an hour, it seems like a minute. But let him sit on a hot stove for a minute — and it's longer than any hour. That's relativity.

Albert Einstein

No man goes before his time — unless the boss leaves early.

Groucho Marx

TINNITUS
...ultra sound.

When you hear the ringing, don't answer it.

I tell ya, life is tough. For years I was getting "ringing in the ears." It's getting worse. Now I'm getting busy signals.

Rodney Dangerfield

Mishearings:
When God gave out heads,
I thought He said beds,
And I asked for a soft one.

When God gave out looks,
I thought He said books,
And I didn't want any.

When God gave out noses,
I thought He said roses,
And I asked for a red one.

When God gave out ears,
I thought He said beers,
And I asked for two big ones.

When God gave out chins,
I thought He said gins,
And I asked for a double.

When God gave out brains,
I thought He said trains,
And I said I'd take the next one.

When God gave out legs,
I thought He said kegs,
So I ordered two fat ones.

Now I'm trying to listen better.

TOASTS
...the only thing that can be eaten or drunk.

Here's champagne to our real friends and real pain to our sham friends.

Here's to your heart, may it last as long as you live.
Here's to your liver, may it live as long as it lasts.

Andrei Gromyko, the Soviet foreign minister, made a completely unintended slip when he proposed a toast to Mrs. Dean Rusk at a Vienna Summit, "I offer a toast to this gracious lady. Up your bottom!" No doubt it was well meant.

I've drunk to your health in company,
I've drunk to your health alone,
I've drunk to your health so many times,
I damn near ruined my own.

Let us drink a toast to the queer old dean.

Rev. William Archibald Spooner
Spoonerism

Addendumb: He is also known for the toast-less question and pun-gent remark — "Is it kisstamary to cuss the bride."

Toastmaster: one who is able to handle his liquor.

Unto our doctors let us drink,
Who cure our chills and ills,
No matter what we really think
About their pills and bills.

Phillip McAllister

TOBACCO
...a habit that lowers one's lungevity.

But can't one lose weight by smoking?
Certainly, give us twenty years and we will take it all off.
The Tobacco Institute

Tobacco is a filthy weed,
That from the devil does proceed;
It drains your purse, it burns your clothes,
And makes a chimney of your nose.

Oliver Wendell Holmes, M.D.

TOOTHPASTE
...an absolute waste of money if your teeth aren't loose.

Electric toothbrush owners are advised to brush twice a day and see their electrician twice a year.

TOUPEE
...a breath of fresh hair.

A man who wears a toupee should take his hat off to no one.
Fred Allen

Things for guys to consider before buying a hairpiece:
Will it appreciate in value?
Is it possible a hairpiece will make me look too good?
Will I be able to handle all the women?
Have I explored all my comb-over options?

David Letterman

Toupee, or not toupee? That is the question:
Whether 'tis nobler in the mind to suffer
The comb and scissors of outrageous barbers,
Or to take arms against the wispy remainders,
And, by shaving, end them — to cut — to snip
No more — and, by a wig, to say we end
The heartache, and the thousand shocks
That scalp is heir to — 'tis a consummation
Devoutly to be wished. To dye — to slick —
To slick! Perchance, to comb — ay, there's the rub;
For in that run of comb through hair what dreams may come,
When we have muffled off our shiny dome,
Must give us pause.

Robert E. Tinsley

TRANQUILIZERS
...little pills that you take to keep from becoming a really big one.

The trouble taking tranquilizers is that you find yourself being nice to
people you dislike.

"Mrs. Smith," said the doctor, "Your husband must have rest and
absolute quiet. Here are some tranquilizer pills — I suggest you take
one every four hours."

TRAVEL
I may be square, but I've been around.

If you don't know where you're going, any road will take you there.

Lewis Carroll
1832-1898

Tip when abroad: In an underdeveloped country, don't drink the water.
In a developed country, don't breathe the air.

Jonathan Raban

I met my wife at the travel bureau.
She was looking for a vacation and I was the last resort.

In the window of a travel agency in Barcelona: "Go away."

One airline security guard searched me so thoroughly, we still write.
Linda Perret

I didn't finish the dinner I was served in the first-class section. The flight attendant said to me, "Finish what's on your tray. Think of all those people who are starving in tourist."

I once went for a job at an airline. The interviewer asked me why I wanted to be a stewardess, and I told her — it would be a great chance to meet men. I was honest about it. She looked at me and said, "But you can meet men anywhere." I said, "Strapped down?"

Terminally ill: the feeling you get when your flight has been cancelled.

When you look like your passport photo, it's time to go home.
Erma Bombeck

It happened at JFK:
My plane from Atlanta arrived late, and I missed the last shuttle to Boston. I indignantly berated the airline clerk about the poor service, complaining that because of the delay I would not get home that night. The clerk explained agreeably that the airline would be happy to pay for a hotel room for me.

Still not satisfied, I told him that it was hours since I'd eaten, and the flight had not been a dinner flight. He handed me a meal ticket, good for whatever I wanted at the terminal restaurant.

Somewhat calmed by now, but still in a complaining mood, I said, "Were it not for your airline, I'd be with my wife tonight." The clerk was quick to reply, "I'm sorry, sir, but we have to draw the line somewhere."
S. Ferraguto

TUBERCULOSIS
Dad always thought laughter was the best medicine, which I guess is why several of us died of tuberculosis.
Jack Handley

Ed Sullivan, closing out his Sunday night TV program, found a few seconds to do a quick public service message, "And now a word about tuberculosis — Good night everybody. Help stamp out TV."

147

TB or not TB, that is congestion.
Consumption be done about it?
Of corpse. Of corpse.
For it's not the cough that carries you off,
It's the coffin they carry you off in.

URINAL
...the one place where all men are peers.

Rick Bayan

Sign in bathrooms:
Our aim is to keep this bathroom clean.
Gentlemen — your aim will help, stand closer. It's shorter than you think.
Ladies — Please remain seated for the entire performance.

As men draw near the common goal,
Can anything be sadder
Than he who, master of his soul,
Is servant to his bladder?

URINALYSIS
...is as good as ours.

I was having breakfast in the hospital, when a nurse came in with a
specimen bottle. When she wasn't looking, I took my apple juice, poured
it into the bottle, and handed it to her. She looked at the bottle and said,
"My, we're looking a little cloudy today, aren't we?" Whereupon I took a
big swig from the bottle and replied, "By George, you're right. Let's run it
through again."

Norman Cousins
Anatomy of an Illness

Peer group: people with weak kidneys.

Some bring their sample in a jar,
Some bring it in a pot,
Some bring a sample hardly ample,
While others bring a lot.

Richard Armout

UROLOGY
It's better to have laughed and leaked then never to have laughed at all.
Merrilyn Belgum

We Treat your Leaks With Tender Loving Care.
Minnesota Radiator Company

Do octogenarians wear boxers or briefs?
"Depends."

This is the incontinence hotline. Can you hold please?
"No! Do you think I'm wearing my lucky underwear?"

Urologist: a pecker checker.

Nocturnal enuresis is a terrible fate,
I try hard to make it, but always I'm late.
My therapist advises, "Don't get so upset."
That's easy for him. I'm the one who gets wet.
E. C. Oliver Jr. R.Ph.

VALUES
He who sees age on the outside of things is doomed to underestimate the value of raisons.

Phillip Jason

Drugs, sex and rock and roll.
What kind of values are these?
I say we go back to the old values:
Wine, women and song.

VEGETARIAN
…a meat defeater.

Vegetarian is an old Indian word meaning "lousy hunter."
Andy Rooney

I came from a poor family. We never had meat at our house. And whenever I would go by a butcher's window, I thought there had been a terrible accident.

Jack Paar

Cannibals are not vegetarians. They are humanitarians.

So these two cannibals are eating a clown and one says, "Does this taste funny to you?"
He answered, "No. Absolutely not. I'm having a ball!"

149

Cannibal converts: those who are fed up with people.

Roots, fruits and nuts,
Muscle, speed and guts,
We're the guys who eat no ham,
We eat no beef, We eat no lamb.
We're vegetarians.
Raw, Raw, Raw!

Bob Cummings

VETERINARIAN
...a dog that was in the army.

News headline: Panda Mating Fails. Veterinarian Takes Over.

Animal husbandry: a wife's nightmare.

Isn't over-pupulation a doggone catastrophe?

VIAGRA (Sildenafil)
...a place out of the blue where one (preferably two) can combine vigor
with a second honeymoon and still not see The Falls.

How is Viagra like Disneyland?
You have to wait an hour for a three minute ride.

Why do they give old men in the nursing home Viagra before they go to
sleep? To keep them from rolling out of bed.

The idea of using Viagra at my age is like erecting a brand new flag pole
in front of a condemned building.

Harvey Korman

VIRUS
...often used by doctors to mean, "Your guess is as good as mine."

Mystery Guest:
Was it the Rotavirus,
The bug that's going around?
Perhaps Rhinovirus
The endangered one?
How about Virus-X

By those who couldn't spell pneumonia?
MRSA, Staph, Strep.
Have you met those guys yet?
I had a little bird
And its name was Enza.
I opened a window
And in-flu-enza.

N.H.

VITAMIN
…what a pharmacist does when a customer knocks.

How was I to know that the B-1 was an airplane?
I thought it was vitamins for the troops.

Ronald Reagan

The pharmacy was out of vitamin B-12, so the patient swallowed a dozen of vitamin B-1.

People crave laughter as if it were an essential amino acid.

Patch Adams M.D.

What are proteins? They are composed of "a mean old acid."

A lusty old lecher named Tim
Decided he needed more vim.
But he took the wrong pill
Which made him quite ill,
And now he's no longer a him.

VOLUNTEER
...a good for nothing?

The only ones among you who will be really happy are those who will have sought and found how to serve.

Albert Schweitzer
1875-1965

I do what I can to help the elderly; after all, I'm going to be old myself some day.

Lillian Carter
1898-1983
At 68, joined Peace Corps

This is a story about people: Everybody, Somebody, Anybody, and Nobody. There was an important job to be done, and Everybody was asked to do it. Everybody was sure Somebody would do it, but Nobody did it. Anybody could have done it, but Nobody did it. Somebody got angry about that because it was Everybody's job. Everybody thought Anybody could do it. Nobody realized Everybody wouldn't do it. In the end, Everybody blamed Somebody when actually Nobody asked Anybody.

WAR AND PEACE
(with apologies to Leo Tolstoy)

When women are depressed, they either eat or go shopping.
Men invade another country.

> Elayne Boosler

The world would not be in such a snarl
If Marx had been Groucho instead of Karl

> Irving Berlin

Frankly, I'd like to see the government get out of war altogether and leave the whole field to private individuals.

> Joseph Heller, 1955
> *Catch-22*

Sometime they'll give a war and nobody will come.

> Carl Sandburg
> 1878-1967

Peace:
To fix the boundaries of earth
Brings nations to the mat.
There are no boundaries of mirth,
Let's all be glad of that.

WARFARIN (Coumadin)
...a D-CONcoction.
Addendumb: Beware of the doctor who tells you to take it with a piece of cheese, unless you want to be anonymous(e).

WEATHER

After three days men grow weary, of a wench, a guest, and weather rainy.
Benjamin Franklin

Tonight's forecast: Dark. Continuing dark throughout the night
and turning to widely scattered light in the morning.
George Carlin

I'm 57 years old, but with the wind-chill factor, I feel like 83.

Market research is about as accurate as my grandmother's big toe was
in predicting the weather.
Garrison Keillor

Weather report from Anchorage Alaska International Airport:
"That's the latest. Now I'll take a leak out the window to see if it's
freezing outside our studio."

Rheumatism: nature's first effort to establish a weather bureau.
My joints are more accurate meteorologists than the weather service.

Meteorologist: A man who can look in a girl's eyes and tell wheather.

The rain, it raineth on the just
And also on the unjust fella:
But chiefly on the just, because
The unjust steals the just's umbrella.
Lord Bowen

WHISKEY

She was only a whiskey maker, but he loved her still.

Whiskey does not make you fat — it makes you lean…
against tables, chairs, floors and walls.

All vodka corrupts. Absolut Vodka corrupts absolutely.
Stefan Kanfer

The Americans are a funny lot. They drink whiskey to keep them warm;
they put some ice in it to make it cool; they put some sugar in it to make
it sweet; and then they put a slice of lemon in it to make it sour. They say,
"Here's to you," and drink it themselves.
B. N. Chakravarty

A Frenchman drinks his native wine,
A German drinks his beer,
An Englishman quaffs 'alf and 'alf
Because it brings good cheer.
The Scotchman drinks his whiskey straight
Because it brings on dizziness.
But we Americans can't choose at all —
So we drink the whole damn business.

WINE
...bottled poetry.

Robert Louis Stevenson

On menu in Swiss restaurant: Our wines leave you nothing to hope for.

I love cooking with wine. Occasionally, I put it in the food.

Robert Morley

There's a new wine for older men. It's called Pinot Moir.
Addendumb: And it's way cheaper than Flomax.

Hangover: the wrath of grapes.

Wine steward: an intoxicaterer offering grape expectations.

Here's to wine, wit and wisdom:
Wine enough to sharpen wit,
Wit enough to give zest to wine
And wisdom enough
To know when I've had enough.

WOMEN
They will never be equal to men until they can walk down the street
with a bald head and a beer gut and still think they're beautiful.

Patty Paul

Build a man a fire and he'll be warm for a day.
Set a man on fire and he'll be warm for the rest of his life.

I am a marvelous housekeeper. Every time I leave a man, I keep his house.

Zsa Zsa Gabor

Women's faults are many, men have only two,
Everything they say and everything they do.

You're not too smart, are you? I like that in a man.

Kathleen Turner
Body Heat

You're handsome and funny,
You're charming and kind,
Your body is stunning,
And so is your mind.
Your talents are many,
Your wardrobe is great'
But nothing surpasses
Your taste in a mate.

Ellen Jackson

WORDS
When I use a word, it means just what I choose it to mean…neither more
nor less.

Lewis Carroll
Of Alice in Wonderland

Addendumb: Flying pigs, buffalo wings, jabberwocky? What a wordo!

A lot of men still don't know that harass isn't two words.

Patricia Schroeder
U.S. Congress, Colorado

The longest word in the English language:
"And now, a word from our sponsor."

2nd longest:
Pneumonoultramicroscopicsilicovolcanoconniosis — Black Lung Disease
If you can pronounce it, you don't have it.

It's good advice to avoid clichés… like the plague.
Addendumb: That's a tough pill to swallow.

London Linguistic Contest: "Some say there is no difference between
COMPLETE and FINISHED. When you marry the right woman,
you are complete. But, if you marry the wrong woman, you are finished.
And when the right one catches you with the wrong one, you are
COMPLETELY FINISHED."

Samsundar Balgobin
From Guyana

155

This I have never understood:
We chop down trees but chop up wood;
We draw down wrath, we draw up wills,
We run down foes, we run up bills;
We eat food up, we down a drink,
Which is a little strange, I think.
We turn down offers, turn up noses —
Just one thought and then this closes:
We should remember, we poor clowns,
That life is full of ups and downs.

Richard Armour

WORK
... the curse of the drinking classes.

Oscar Wilde

When the boss tells a joke, he who laughs — lasts.

Tell your boss what you really think of him and the truth will set you free.

At job interview: Does the company offer an employee health plan?
Yes, we plan to allow you to work as long as you're healthy.

Dan Piraro

You can tell a company by the men it keeps.

W. A. Clarke

There is a dangerous virus being passed around electronically, orally,
and by hand. This virus is called Worm Overload Recreational Killer
(WORK).

If you receive WORK from any of your colleagues, your boss, or
anyone else via any means, do not touch it. This virus will wipe out your
private life completely.

If you should come in contact with WORK, put your jacket on and
take two good friends to the nearest grocery store. Purchase the antidote
known as Work Isolating Neutralizer Extract (WINE) or Bothersome
Employer Elimination Rebooter (BEER).

Use the antidote repeatedly until WORK is completely eliminated
from your system.

You should forward this warning to five friends. If you do not have five
friends, you have already been infected and WORK is controlling your life.

Addendumb: People who work in glass offices should never scratch where
it itches and avoid getting stoned.

WRINKLES
...the service stripes of life.

They should merely indicate where smiles have been.
Mark Twain

They're something other people have. You have character lines.

She tried to improve her wrinkles by rubbing her body with Vitamin A, D, and E. It worked, but she kept rolling out of bed.

WRITING
...Authoritis.

It is simply thinking through my fingers.
Isaac Asimov

I've written several children's books. I didn't mean to. They just turned out that way.

Your manuscript is both good and original. But the part that is good is not original, and the part that is original is not good.
Samuel Johnson
1709-1784

She began writing as soon as she left college, and within six months, she sold several articles — her watch, her overcoat, her typewriter.

Every time you make a typo you lose, and the errorists win.

Some books are to be tasted, others to be swallowed, and some few to be chewed and digested.
Sir Francis Bacon
"Sir, have you ever had to eat your own words?"

"Brevity is the soul of wit," they say. And it's the body and soul of lingerie.

It has often been said, "There's so much to be read,
You never can cram all those thoughts in your head.
So the writer who breeds more words than he needs
Is making a chore for the reader who reads.
That's why my belief is: the briefer the brief is,
The greater the sigh of the reader's relief is."
Dr. Seuss

X-RAY
...belly vision.

I got a chest X-ray last month and they found a spot on my lung.
Fortunately it was barbecue sauce. I also said, "I had onions on my liver."

Anyone who says he can see through women is missing a lot.
Groucho Marx

An eager inventor named Jones
Was reduced to loud sobbing and moans.
He'd devised X-ray glasses
To study clothed lasses,
But all he could see were their bones.
Issac Asimov

YAWN
...an honest opinion openly expressed.
Addendumb: It's OK, you're almost through.

YOUTH
You grow up the day you have the first real laugh — at yourself.
Ethel Barrymore

The heart is the real Fountain of Youth.
Mark Twain

The young don't know what to do, while the old can't do what they know.

Never wear a backward baseball cap to a job interview unless you're
applying for the job of an umpire.

Today's kids have everything. My son has his own TV, VCR, DVD,
CD player, cell phone, and refrigerator in his room. When I punish him,
I have to send him to my room.

Can young people wear their pants any lower? Their waistbands are
now at approximately knee level. Where will this trend end? The shins?
The feet? Will young people eventually detach themselves from their
pants altogether and just drag them along behind, connected to their
ankles by a belt?
Dave Barry

ZZZZZ

You go to bed; you can't sleep yet;
You decide to count a couple of sheep yet;
Well, you count ten; you count twenty;
You count more, you count plenty.
You find more sheep than you expected,
But there isn't one that you neglected.
You waited while they stopped to browse yet;
You even counted stray cows yet;
You threw in lambs, you threw in rabbits;
You threw in goats with nervous habits.
Your head aches; your eyes humming —
And what thanks do you get?
The sheep keep coming.

Samuel Hoffenstein

Appendix
(Of another sort)

The Association For Applied And Therapeutic Humor (AATH) is dedicated to educating health care, business and education professionals about the values and therapeutic uses of humor and laughter. The organization also offers research on humor and laughter, supports innovative programs which incorporate the therapeutic use of humor, and serves as a clearinghouse of information on humor and laughter as they relate to well-being. www.aath.org

TO CONTACT AUTHOR
nhoesl@yahoo.com www.laughterdoc.com

Special thanks to Pharmacy Times for use of the smiling mortar and pestle.